Amanda Pozos Ravelo
Víctor Manuel Hernández Uz
Rosío de la C Estrada Fonseca

Diabetic Neuropathy

Amanda Pozos Ravelo
Víctor Manuel Hernández Uz
Rosío de la C Estrada Fonseca

Diabetic Neuropathy

Assessment of diabetic patient care for diagnosis and treatment

ScienciaScripts

Imprint
Any brand names and product names mentioned in this book are subject to trademark, brand or patent protection and are trademarks or registered trademarks of their respective holders. The use of brand names, product names, common names, trade names, product descriptions etc. even without a particular marking in this work is in no way to be construed to mean that such names may be regarded as unrestricted in respect of trademark and brand protection legislation and could thus be used by anyone.

Cover image: www.ingimage.com

This book is a translation from the original published under ISBN 978-613-8-98501-3.

Publisher:
Sciencia Scripts
is a trademark of
Dodo Books Indian Ocean Ltd. and OmniScriptum S.R.L publishing group

120 High Road, East Finchley, London, N2 9ED, United Kingdom
Str. Armeneasca 28/1, office 1, Chisinau MD-2012, Republic of Moldova, Europe
Printed at: see last page
ISBN: 978-620-7-94236-7

Contents

Authors

Dr. Amanda Pozas Ravelo
Dr. in Medicine First Degree Specialist in MGI
Dr. Víctor Manuel Hernández Uz
Dr in Medicine First Degree Specialist in MGI
Rosío de la C. Estrada Fonseca.
Licentiate in Nursing. Master's Degree in Comprehensive Child Care. Assistant Professor.

Research Attaché

SUMMARY

Diabetic neuropathy is the leading complication of diabetes. In order to evaluate the comprehensive care of diabetic patients, in terms of early detection and treatment of diabetic neuropathy, an investigation was carried out in health systems and services through a descriptive observational study from September/2021 to June/2023. From the Santo Domingo health area, 35 doctors and 54 patients with diabetic neuropathy were selected by intentional sampling. By means of a questionnaire for professionals, an interview, a general and neurological physical examination, complementary tests and a review of the patients' medical records, information was obtained for the evaluation of some of the components of the structure and process of the Diabetic Patient Comprehensive Care Programme. 50.0% of the patients presented symmetrical and distal polyneuropathy, 25.9% being over 70 years of age. A total of 87.0% were type 2 diabetics and 40.7% had been diagnosed between 10 and 15 years previously. There was a lack of quality in the follow-up and control in all the indicators studied, particularly in the physical examination (51.0%) and the establishment of a correct diagnostic impression (49.1%). 65.7% of the professionals had a high need for knowledge about neuropathy and 77.1% had difficulties in diagnosis. In the health area, the design of a professional training programme on diabetic neuropathy and the inclusion of all medical professionals, regardless of their degree of specialisation, is urgently required.

1 INTRODUCTION

Diabetes Mellitus is a condition with a high incidence and prevalence in the world population, which is also increasing in alarming proportions, acquiring the characteristics of a pandemic, as it is one of the pathologies that generates the greatest disability and mortality, especially in the elderly, occupying a large part of the health resources in all countries.

Diabetes Mellitus is characterised by metabolic disturbances of multiple aetiologies due to chronic hyperglycaemia and disturbances in carbohydrate, fat and protein metabolism, resulting from defects in insulin secretion, insulin action or both. [1]

The World Health Organisation currently estimates that some 422 million people worldwide suffer from diabetes, a figure that is likely to double in the next 20 years. [2] Of these, approximately 30 million are in the Americas.[3] Hence, according to estimates, the global prevalence of diabetes mellitus, which was 2.8% in 2000, will increase to 10.4% by 2040. This phenomenon is attributed, in addition to genetic factors, to the fact that humans have changed their lifestyles. [4]

The International Diabetes Federation states in the ninth edition of its atlas that 8.3% of the world's population has Diabetes Mellitus and this figure is projected to rise to more than 592 million cases, an increase of 55% (also taking into account that there are at least 175 million people with the disease who are undiagnosed). The largest number of cases is in the Western Pacific region with 138 million, followed by South-East Asia with a total of 72 million and Europe with 56 million people with the disease. [5]

In 2016, diabetes was the direct cause of 1.6 million deaths, with a predominance of females with 124 812 more deaths than males, mainly in the age group of patients aged 70 years and older. South-East Asia was the region with the highest number of diabetes deaths, followed by the Americas and the Western Pacific. The regions with the lowest numbers of diabetes deaths were the Eastern Mediterranean, Africa and Europe. [6]

In Spain, there is a prevalence of 13.8% in people over 18 years of age, and it is estimated that the complications of Diabetes Mellitus generate between 7 and 12 deaths per 100,000 inhabitants, accounting for 10% of hospital admissions. [7]

In the United States, 10.25% of the population is affected by diabetes and an average of 30 million people are still undiagnosed, making it the seventh leading cause of death in the population. [8]

In Central and South America there are 29.6 million people with diabetes and it is projected that there will be 48.8 million by 2040, representing one of the largest increases in prevalence in the world. In South America alone, Brazil documented 11.9 million people with diabetes mellitus, Colombia 2.1 million, Argentina 1.6 million and Chile 1.3 million. [9-12]

The problem is magnified by the fact that at least one third of people with diabetes mellitus in Latin America are unaware of their condition, which challenges the screening programme and complicates the implementation of care, control and prevention strategies. [13]

This has a high economic impact, such that in 2016 most countries had spent between 5-20% of their total health budget on diabetes-related expenditures[1,4] , which in absolute terms is about $750 billion annually and with the potential to increase by 19.0% over the next 25 years. [4]

Cuba is not far from this situation, so much so that the 49th edition of the Statistical Yearbook of Health indicates that in 2020 the prevalence of Diabetes Mellitus was 66.7 per 1 000 inhabitants, including all ages; likewise, 2 313 deaths from this disease were reported, for a mortality rate of 20.6 per 100 000 inhabitants, making it the eighth leading cause of death in the country.

The province of Villa Clara reported a prevalence of 66.9 patients with Diabetes Mellitus per 1000 inhabitants and a total of 129 deaths, representing a crude mortality rate of 16.6 per 100 000 inhabitants, surpassed only by Havana, Santiago de Cuba, Camagüey and Granma in that order. [14]

In the municipality of Santo Domingo there is a prevalence of 2464 patients with type 2 diabetes mellitus, of whom 1543 are female, with six deaths reported in 2020, representing a mortality rate of 0.12 per 1000 inhabitants, so that these data are closely related to the provincial and national average. [15]

Unfortunately, a high proportion of diabetic patients do not follow a good behaviour, which leads to complications that constantly require outpatient and inpatient health services. The most common complications are retinopathies, retinopathies, retinopathies and retinopathy.

neuropathies, nephropathies, diabetic foot and autonomic cardiac, gastrointestinal, genitourinary and ischaemic complications. [16]

Diabetic neuropathy ranks first among the complications of diabetes, appearing at any stage of the disease, but is more frequent in the late stages. Furthermore, diabetic neuropathy can occur in any patient with both type 1 and type 2 diabetes mellitus. This complication can begin suddenly or gradually, and resolve quickly or have a chronic, insidious and progressive course. It usually affects mainly the peripheral nerves, but also the cerebral cortex and, in early cases of dementia of diabetic origin, it can involve any structure of the nervous system with a large number of clinical manifestations. [16,17]

In the literature, reported prevalences of patients with diabetic neuropathy range from 10-90%, so that approximately 30 million patients worldwide suffer from some form of diabetic neuropathy and it is also a direct cause of 50-75% of non-traumatic amputations, making this condition a major public health problem. [17]

Diabetic neuropathy is present in 40-50% of patients 10 years after the onset of the disease. Its prevalence increases with the time of evolution of the disease and with the age of the patient, its extent and severity being related to the degree and duration of hyperglycaemia. Signs and symptoms of diabetic neuropathy are manifested by the diabetic patient in only 10-15% of all cases and, therefore, the lowest prevalence figures are obtained when the study is carried out exclusively on the basis of clinical anamnesis data.[17-20]

Its prevalence is difficult to establish due to the absence of unified diagnostic criteria, the multiplicity of diagnostic methods and the heterogeneity of clinical forms. Its evolution and severity correlate with the duration of the disease and poor metabolic control.[18,19]

Several authors also agree that diabetic neuropathy is a complication that is diagnosed and treated late; unfortunately, our country is not exempt from this problem; this is largely due to the lack of knowledge on the part of professionals about diagnostic criteria, preventive measures and specific treatments, the lack of time available during medical consultations and, finally, the lack of sufficient studies based on population-based research.[17,18,20-22]

This manifestation of microvascular damage affects the quality of life and life expectancy of people with diabetes and it is the responsibility of the healthcare team to be aware of it, to detect it and to implement rational measures for its treatment.[20]

In Cuba, since 1975, the National Institute of Endocrinology developed a National Programme of Comprehensive Care for Diabetics, setting the goal of reducing mortality from diabetes by 15% in the population aged 15-64 years by the year 2000 and subsequently ratifying the decision to prioritise this programme, Even in the difficult economic conditions of the so-called Special Period of the 1990s, the National Institute of Endocrinology and the National Diabetes Commission were assigned the task of promoting its progress in the context of the development of the Non-Communicable Diseases Programme.[23]

The daily actions of primary health care professionals play a fundamental role in the programme, who, from their position, are the first link in the prevention and early detection of this unfortunate disease, as they are primarily responsible for the educational process that is the cornerstone of treatment. Education, as well as comprehensive care for people with diabetes mellitus, is thus the cornerstone of prevention.[23-25]

Promoting the screening for diabetic neuropathy in primary care is essential to reduce the risk of disability as well as to improve the quality of life of diabetic patients, which is closely related to the goals of the National Programme of Care for People with Diabetes Mellitus established in 1996[23] , where the level of training and education of doctors with respect to current knowledge, the availability of increasingly effective drugs for treatment, prevention of complications and strategies for metabolic control will have a positive impact on the natural history of diabetes mellitus and neuropathy as one of its chronic complications.

We are therefore motivated to carry out this research in order to answer the following question:

Scientific Problem: What are the aspects that affect the care of diabetic patients, in terms of diagnosis and treatment of diabetic neuropathy, in the health area of Santo Domingo from September/2021 to June/2023?

2 OBJECTIVES

1. To describe the sample of patients according to clinical-epidemiological variables of interest and type of neuropathy.
2. Determine the quality of follow-up and monitoring of diabetic patients.
3. To identify the knowledge needs on diabetic neuropathy in medical professionals according to their degree of specialisation.
4. Identify the thematic clusters concerned.

3 THEORETICAL FRAMEWORK

I.Diabetes Mellitus. General.

Despite the recent epidemic of diabetes, this disease has accompanied mankind since our earliest historical memories, as it was already mentioned by the Egyptians in the Ebers papyrus (1550 BC), a compilation of medical texts describing the diseases known at that time. Later, the Greek Areteus of Cappadocia (30 to 90 A.D.) gave it the name of diabetes, which means siphon, portraying the increase in the frequency of urination or polyuria, but it was not until 1679 that Thomas Willis made a masterly description of diabetes, and since then its symptoms have been recognised as a clinical entity and it was given the name of Diabetes Mellitus (honey flavour). [26,27]

Diabetes mellitus is currently considered a syndrome characterised by chronic hyperglycaemia due to defects in insulin secretion, insulin action or both; there are also alterations in the metabolism of proteins and lipids. This condition is associated, in the long term, with microcirculation damage to organs such as the retina, kidneys and large blood vessels of the heart, brain and lower limbs; it also affects the peripheral and autonomic nervous system. [28-30]

The conception of diabetes as a chronic disease and its trajectory has facilitated the development of means and procedures of intervention for primary prevention, early detection and treatment (curative, damage limitation, replacement, palliative or rehabilitative).[30]

Therefore, patients with diabetes mellitus require continuous medical care, but they also need proper education to manage the disease, prevent acute complications, reduce the risk of chronic complications and, ultimately, increase quality of life. [22,30]

Complications of diabetes can be divided into acute and chronic. Within the first group we find those that require emergency treatment, they are often the form in which the disease debuts and it is mainly type 1 diabetics who develop them most frequently. [5,9,17] These include diabetic ketoacidosis, hyperglycaemic hyperosmolar state, lactic acidosis and hypoglycaemia (which is considered a complication of treatment). On the other hand, the most frequent chronic complications are diabetic retinopathy, diabetic nephropathy, coronary artery disease, arterial hypertension and diabetic neuropathy. [22,30,31]

Other diabetic complications include bacterial and fungal infections such as osteomyelitis (bacterial bone infection), vulvovaginal and oral candidiasis. [22,31-34]

As the prevalence of diabetes mellitus continues to increase, we will witness an increase in the complications associated with the underlying disease, which have a substantial impact on the quality of life of the individuals who suffer from them. Diabetes Mellitus is characterised by a strong predisposition to compromise microvascular territories; diabetic neuropathy is the most faithful exposition of this damage. It is responsible for causing excess morbidity and mortality and is accompanied by considerable economic, family and social costs. [34-37]

II. Diabetic neuropathy.

Peripheral nerve disorders caused by diabetes mellitus as a secondary abnormality have been identified for more than a century, although the symptoms were known long before. Reports of diabetic neuropathy were mainly from pathological work on necropsy tissue or amputated limbs, in which the presence or degradation of peripheral nerve fibres related to the degenerative process of diabetes was established. From the mid-20th century onwards, clinical and epidemiological research began to provide detailed information on the prevalence and clinical heterogeneity, as well as the complex pathogenic mechanisms of diabetic neuropathy. [38,39]

Definition.

It is now accepted that nervous system damage in people with diabetes is the most prevalent and earliest-onset microangiopathic manifestation. Current studies indicate that diabetic neuropathy appears incipiently not only in patients with long-standing diabetes, but also in newly diagnosed patients and even in those who meet the criteria for non-diabetic dysglycaemia and, even more so, if they are accompanied by alterations in lipid metabolism and arterial hypertension. [40]

Diabetic neuropathy is defined as the set of symptoms and signs of peripheral and autonomic nervous system dysfunction caused by Diabetes Mellitus, after other causes of neuropathy have been excluded. Other authors define it as peripheral nerve damage, primarily of the sensory type, which initially occurs in the distal region of the lower extremities attributable to diabetes mellitus and is found in two out of three diabetics at the time of clinical examination. [39,40]

It should be taken into account that this pathology is a diagnosis of exclusion and it is estimated that it is present in 10% to 90% of patients with diabetes, while electrophysiological studies show alterations in almost 100% of them [40].

Diabetic neuropathy involves 50-75% of non-traumatic lower limb amputation. The progression of neuropathy is dependent on the degree of glycaemic control in Type 1 and Type 2 diabetes. The causes are multifactorial, and are related to hyperglycaemia and insulin deficiency; although in most patients, neuropathy is of unknown or idiopathic cause. Its genesis is related to complex metabolic, vascular, neurotrophic and autoimmune interactions that lead to inflammation, malfunction and ultimately permanent damage to peripheral nerve fibres. [28,29] Diabetes duration, age, smoking, hypertension and dyslipidaemia are also risk factors for diabetic neuropathy. Other causes include genetic factors, chemical agents such as chemotherapy drugs and HIV. [41,42]

Diabetic neuropathy affects all peripheral nerves, damaging motor neuron fibres and autonomic nerves. Therefore, it can potentially affect all organs and systems as they are all innervated. A patient may have sensory-motor and autonomic neuropathy or any other combination. [43]

Symptoms vary depending on the nerves affected and usually occur gradually over years. [18]

Neuropathy is recognised as the main cause of the "diabetic foot", although it must also be acknowledged that its relevance clearly exceeds the involvement of the lower limbs. [40,43]

In addition to the involvement of the patients' limbs and the Autonomic Nervous System lesions that affect all the organs of the economy that receive this type of innervation, it is important to recognise damage to the Central Nervous System, although its study is not systematised like the previous ones. Diabetic polyneuropathy should be understood as a heterogeneous microvascular disorder comprising a wide range of abnormalities that may be asymptomatic, oligosymptomatic, or on the contrary have clinical manifestations (usually in advanced stages) with a limiting effect on quality of life. [44]

One of the aspects to be highlighted is that diabetic polyneuropathy is usually diagnosed late, a situation that can be explained by its initial symptoms, until it reaches severe deterioration, as well as by the lack of a search for it. Given the lack of unified criteria for diagnosis, the incorrect performance of the neurological physical examination in medical consultations, as well as the poor relevance given to neuropathic symptoms, there are no reliable figures regarding its prevalence. [39-42]

This manifestation of microvascular damage affects the quality of life and life expectancy of people with diabetes and it is the responsibility of the healthcare team to be aware of it, to detect it and to implement rational measures for its treatment. The wide universe of this complication makes it necessary for the medical professional caring for people with diabetes to have an open and integrative view of it. This situation justifies the emphasis on the implementation of the corresponding measures for the early diagnosis and treatment of each of the conditions or variables that are associated with the affectation of the nervous system. [39]

Pathogenesis.

The pathogenesis of this complication has not yet been fully elucidated; the multi-causality of this complication is accepted and it is considered to be the result of several combined mechanisms that concur over time. It is still not possible to define the predominant element that triggers and/or perpetuates the initial functional and subsequent anatomical alterations of the nerve damage in the diabetic environment, but it is accepted that hyperglycaemia is a factor of primary relevance in the genesis of neuropathic involvement, triggering the different metabolic pathways involved. This reasoning is used to emphasise the need to optimise glycaemic control, which is essential for any type of aetiopathogenic or symptomatic intervention. In addition, it is now accepted that other metabolic factors such as lipid alterations have a deleterious effect on nerve structure, as do genetic determinants of individual susceptibility, arterial hypertension and hyperhomocysteinemia. [40]

In diabetes there is a complex interplay between metabolic, vascular and hormonal factors involved in the balance between damage and repair of nerve fibres in favour of the former. The distal sensory and autonomic fibres are the ones to be preferentially affected, leading to the progressive loss of sensation that precedes the clinical manifestations of diabetic neuropathy. [44]

The specific mechanism by which the sustained hyperglycaemic state and cardiovascular factors predispose to microvascular disease is not well understood at present. However, there are several theories about the metabolic factors involved including the following:

> Accumulation of advanced glycation end products.

> Sorbitol accumulation.

> Disruption of the hexosamine pathway.

> Disruption of the protein kinase C pathway.

> Activation of the poly (ADP-ribose) polymerase pathway.

> Increased oxidative stress. [41]

<u>Accumulation of advanced glycation products.</u>

Deposits of advanced glycation products cause damage to peripheral nerves as well as to myelin basic protein and proteolipids. Myelin undergoing modification is identified by macrophages that bind to specific receptors for advanced glycation products and form cross-links between proteins, leading to segmental demyelination. Tubulin, neurofilaments and actin are also affected by glycosylation, resulting in conduction slowing, atrophy and axonal degeneration. [40]

<u>Sorbitol pathway.</u>

Intracellular glucose is predominantly metabolised by phosphorylation and subsequent glycolysis, but when it is increased, it is biotransformed to sorbitol. The impact on diabetic complications is through accumulation of the products formed (reduced adenine dinucleotide adenine dinucleotide and fructose) and compensatory depletion of osmolytes (myoinositol and taurine).

Myoinositol depletion is involved in the early modification of nerve conduction velocity as it is associated with altered cellular redux potential, phosphoinositide metabolism and reduced Na+/K+ ATPase activity. [40,41]

<u>Hexosamine pathway.</u>

The upregulation of this pathway contributes to the stimulation of the expression of genes such as transforming growth factor (TGF) and plasminogen activator inhibitor-1 (PAI-1) involved in the induction of lipid-mediated insulin resistance and hyperglycaemia. [40]

<u>Protein Kinase C activation.</u>

Protein kinase C is involved in different signal transduction processes and in the regulation of gene expression such as extracellular matrix proteins (fibronectin and collagen type IV), PAI-1 and TGF-p and its receptor. In addition, it affects the manufacture of vasoactive substances, stimulates endothelin expression and reduces nitric oxide production, leading to decreased blood flow mainly to the retina, peripheral nerves and kidney.

<u>Poly (adp-ribose) polymerase.</u>

Poly (ADP-ribose) polymerase is a nuclear enzyme that is activated in response to high glucose levels, whose function is DNA repair. Excess activation of poly (ADP-ribose) polymerase results in increased free radical formation, alterations in gene transcription, increased protein kinase C activity and the formation of advanced glycosylation products.

Oxidative stress.

Oxidative stress is caused by increased production of reactive oxygen species and decreased antioxidant defence systems caused by hyperglycaemia. Oxidative modification of macromolecules and transcription factor (NFkB) activation lead to altered gene expression leading to the development of diabetic complications. [40,41]

The analysis of all these pathways, in addition to trying to define and complete the knowledge of the mechanisms involved in diabetic neuropathy, has the fundamental objective of finding drugs that can have a positive impact on it. [40]

Risk factors.

In the medical literature, various risk factors for the development of diabetic neuropathy have been postulated, including the age of the patient and the age of diabetes, as well as poor glycaemic and metabolic control. Other factors include dyslipidaemia, high blood pressure, obesity, smoking and alcoholism. [42,43]

Age.

Several groups of researchers have shown that age exerts an independent effect on diabetic neuropathy, leading to a progressive increase in its prevalence for approximately every decade of life. Nervous system disturbances are seen as a late complication of the disease, thus diabetic neuropathy is most common in diabetics over 50 years of age, rare in those under 30 years of age and very rare in childhood. [39,40]

Time course of diabetes mellitus.

The duration of diabetes is an important and well-recognised risk factor for diabetic neuropathy. Most of the literature has reported its presence more than 10 years into the course of diabetes, however it is established that the first signs and symptoms of neuropathic involvement may appear during the first 5 years of the disease. [40]

Estimates of the incidence and prevalence of distal symmetric polyneuropathy vary greatly, but evidence from several cohorts suggests that it occurs in at least 20% of people with type 1 diabetes after 20 years of disease duration and may be present in at least 10-15% of newly diagnosed patients with type 2 diabetes, with rates increasing to 50% after 10 years of disease duration and accounts for approximately 30% of hospitalised patients with diabetes. [44]

Glycaemic and metabolic control.

Optimal diabetes control, including HbA1c less than 7%, blood pressure less than 130/80 mmHg and lipids at therapeutic target, reduces the incidence of neuropathy, the main risk factor for foot ulcers, by up to 59%. [40.43]

It is proposed that in patients with type 1 diabetes mellitus the development of confirmed neuropathy is approximately 50-60% in patients without adequate metabolic control, compared to less than 10% of tightly controlled patients, indicating that long-term tight metabolic control may reduce the prevalence despite a long-standing course. [44]

Hyperglycaemia is another risk factor, its importance has been documented in both type 1 and type 2 diabetes mellitus. It has been estimated that each 1% increase in

HbA1c increases the risk of developing symmetrical and distal polyneuropathy by 10 to 15%. Adequate and timely control of hyperglycaemia decreases the onset of neuropathy by 60% at 5 years. Even glucose intolerance in the absence of frank diabetes is a risk factor for neuropathy. [41-45]

<u>Dyslipidaemia and obesity.</u>

Several studies show that obesity and dyslipidaemia are important risk factors for early diabetic neuropathy, independent of glycaemic control. Furthermore, they correlated significantly with small fibre integrity, while glucose control correlated more closely with large myelinated fibre function. [40,41]

In type 2 diabetes mellitus, the use of fibrates and statins significantly reduces the incidence of neuropathy over 5 years. Similarly, a significant reduction in the rate of lower limb amputations following treatment with fenofibrate has been demonstrated [40].

Obesity has been identified as a risk factor for diabetic neuropathy. In the general population, age $\geq$40 years, obesity and the presence of at least 2 cardiovascular risk factors (elevated triglycerides or plasma glucose, reduced HDL, increased waist circumference and hypertension) increase the likelihood of peripheral neuropathy. Morbidly obese subjects have been found to exhibit features of dysfunction more specifically on small nerve fibres. [40-45]

<u>Arterial Hypertension.</u>

Hypertension is another risk factor for developing diabetic neuropathy, but there is a difference between the two types of diabetes. In type 1 diabetes, data have identified hypertension as the strongest predictor of diabetic neuropathy, increasing the relative risk approximately fourfold over a 6-year period. In contrast, studies in patients with type 2 diabetes report that tight blood pressure control does not reduce the deterioration of the pathology. [42-45]

<u>Smoking.</u>

In people without diabetes, cigarette smoking has been positively associated with elevated HbA1c levels. Smoking is associated with oxidative stress, systemic inflammation and endothelial dysfunction and may increase the risk of nerve damage through these pathways in association with other metabolic factors, and may induce neuropathy through hypoxaemia and microvascular insufficiency. [40,42]

<u>Alcohol consumption.</u>

Some studies have reported an association between distal symmetrical polyneuropathy and alcohol consumption. However, it can be difficult to differentiate between distal symmetrical polyneuropathy with alcohol as a risk factor and alcoholic neuropathy in a person with diabetes. Alcoholic neuropathy presents as a distal, symmetrical sensory-motor neuropathy. Electrophysiological and pathological findings indicate mainly an axonal neuropathy with reduced nerve fibre densities. [40]

Clinical forms of diabetic neuropathy.

The clinical presentation of diabetic neuropathy is very heterogeneous, as it can affect different parts of the nervous system, both in a focal and diffuse manner, which makes its clinical manifestations highly variable. Usually, these clinical manifestations are classified into different clinical syndromes: symmetric distal polyneuropathy and autonomic neuropathy are the most frequent forms; other less frequent presentations are cranial and peripheral mononeuropathy, lumbar or thoracic polyradiculopathy and mononeuropathy multiplex. [31,40]

There are multiple international classifications of diabetic neuropathy. The latest edition of the ALAD Guidelines on the Diagnosis, Management and Treatment of Type 2 Diabetes Mellitus proposes the following classification according to the level of nerve fibre involvement: [9,34]

1- Somatic neuropathy.

J Distal symmetric polyneuropathy.

J Mixed neuropathy.

2- Autonomic neuropathy.

J Cardiovascular.

- Reduced heart rate variability.
- Tachycardia at rest.
- Orthostatic hypotension.
- Sudden death (malignant arrhythmia).

J Gastrointestinal.

- Diabetic gastroparesis (gastropathy).
- Diabetic enteropathy (diarrhoea).
- Colonic hypomotility (constipation).

J Urogenital or Genitourinary.

- Diabetic cystopathy (neurogenic bladder).
- Erectile dysfunction.
- Female sexual dysfunction. [31]

Distal polyneuropathy is the most frequent form of presentation of diabetic neuropathies, accounting for more than 75% of them, which is why diabetic neuropathy and distal symmetrical polyneuropathy are often equated [43-45].

There is evidence that distal symmetric polyneuropathy, especially the painful subtype of small fibre neuropathy, may be present in 8% of newly diagnosed diabetic patients and more than 50% in long term diabetic patients. In addition, 10-30% of subjects with impaired glucose tolerance, pre-diabetes or metabolic syndrome have it. Thus, distal symmetric polyneuropathy is the most important cause of foot ulceration and is also a prerequisite for the development of Charcot neuroarthropathy.

The predominant involvement is of the sensory fibres, of the axonal type, which often manifests itself through a painful neuropathy, as the thin fibres are involved. The clinical and neurophysiological diagnosis will be mainly directed towards this form of neuropathy. In general, motor involvement is less relevant, but there are some pure motor sensory pictures. [31]

Clinical manifestations.

Involvement of the somatic nervous system is the most common form of distal symmetrical polyneuropathy; its involvement results in the loss of its protective functions and is responsible for around 60% of foot lesions. Sensory dysfunction or injury with a minor motor component usually predominates, however, the concept of sensory-motor neuropathy should be maintained for its clinical and therapeutic relevance. [40]

It is important to consider the probable simultaneous involvement of the autonomic nervous system, which, due to its anatomical characteristics of fine fibres and amyelinic fibres, may be altered at multiple levels in early stages, known as mixed neuropathy. [46-49]

Thus, cardiac, genitourinary, gastrointestinal autonomic damage, impaired perception of hypoglycaemia symptoms, impaired sweating (diabetic anhidrosis) and taste as well as lack of pupillary accommodation can be observed. [44]

So the early signs of diabetic polyneuropathy reflect the gradual loss of integrity of both large and small myelinated and unmyelinated nerve fibres:

J Loss of vibratory sensation and impaired proprioception reflect impairment of the large nerve fibre.

J Deterioration of pain, light touch and temperature are secondary to the loss of small fibres. [40]

Painful diabetic neuropathy affects approximately 25% of diabetic patients, treated with insulin and/or oral hypoglycaemic agents, and is characterised by a symmetrical distal neuropathy associated with chronic pain. It is usually vascular in cause, resulting in primary sensory nerve damage due to neuronal hypoxia and nutrient deficiency. [40-44]

Pain is the most relevant symptom and has various characteristics, it is described as burning, shooting, tingling or electric and is exacerbated at night. In the most painful forms, there is an increased sensitivity of the skin in the affected area that makes the rubbing of clothes or sheets intolerable. In addition, it may be accompanied by paraesthesias, exaggerated response to painful stimuli (hyperalgesia) and contact-evoked pain (allodynia). It can also interfere with daily activities, lead to disability, psychosocial impairment and reduced quality of life.

The onset is usually bilateral in toes and feet. In cases of asymmetric origin, progression is towards bilaterality. It may gradually progress to calves and knees, in which case patients may note algic symptoms and/or paraesthesias jointly in hands and feet; sock or glove-sock sensory deficits and loss or decrease of the Achilles reflex are characteristic, although some patients with involvement of only small nerve fibres may have preserved reflexes and vibratory sensitivity. Allodynia and hyperalgesia are less common. [44]

Other symptoms that can be found are vascular claudication, dysautonomic signs (abnormal skin colouring and temperature, sweating), depression and anxiety, sleep disorders, etc. In painful diabetic neuropathy, sensory manifestations are predominant, and in most cases symptoms are mild or absent and the presence of neuropathy is detected at the time of physical examination.[46] In early stages it reveals inhibition or loss of Achilles reflexes, impaired vibratory sensation and distal symmetrical loss of skin sensation, including temperature, fine touch and pain. The deficit is usually restricted to the legs. In more advanced cases there may also be loss of patellar reflexes and altered vibration, joint position, deep pain sensation in the legs and feet and occasionally in the forearms and hands. [46-49]

In many cases distal motor involvement occurs resulting in atrophy of the intrinsic foot muscles, imbalance between strength in the toe extensors and flexors and extensive loss of reflexes. This leads to chronic metatarsal-falangeal flexion (claw-toe deformity) which shifts weight to the metatarsal heads and results in the formation of corns which may develop fissures, infections and ulcers. [49]

The presence of foot ulcers is the ultimate expression of neuropathic involvement, determined by sensory, motor and autonomic disturbances, which are an indicator of advanced neuropathy. [40]

Diabetic autonomic neuropathy can affect various organs and systems, cardiovascular, gastrointestinal, genitourinary, adrenal, sweat glands and pupillary, among others. It usually manifests in long-standing diabetics, but can occur early in the course of the disease, sometimes within a year of type 2 diabetes mellitus, and is usually correlated with the presence of distal sensory polyneuropathy. The prevalence of autonomic neuropathy, detected by heart rate interval studies, is as high as 25%, but with low numbers of symptomatic patients. Cardiovascular autonomic neuropathy results in impaired heart rate control and dysfunction of central and peripheral vascular mechanisms, with increased heart rate and heart rate variability being characteristic signs. Several studies suggest increased mortality and reduced life expectancy in patients with cardiovascular autonomic impairment. Autonomic neuropathy also explains the existence of some silent myocardial infarctions. Exercise intolerance is another common symptom, due to impaired cardiac ejection fraction and dysfunction of peripheral muscle supply mechanisms. Postural hypotension, defined as a decrease of more than 30 mmHg on standing, with orthostatic dizziness and syncopal sensation, is common due to impaired sympathetic innervation. Postural hypotension, together with impaired cardiovascular reflexes, are the key to the diagnosis of autonomic neuropathy. [40-45]

Gastrointestinal manifestations include gastropathy, which may be present in 75% of patients. Symptoms include early satiety, nausea, vomiting and epigastric pain. Vomiting may show retained food up to 8-12 hours post ingestion. There are also intestinal transit disorders, which are an expression of visceral autonomic neuropathy, such as diarrhoea or constipation, which have a prevalence of up to 35%. They usually present with nocturnal diarrhoea lasting hours or days, alternating with constipation, which may also frequently occur as an independent symptom. Faecal incontinence and dysphagia are other symptoms, which may occur in the context of gastrointestinal autonomic involvement. [40,42]

Erectile dysfunction can be found in up to 50% of male diabetic patients, especially at older ages, and is related to neuropathic, vascular, metabolic and psychogenic factors.

Sensory bladder disorders, with a neurogenic bladder, can be found in 37-59% of patients, leading to an increased threshold for voiding reflex, with increased retention capacity, which can lead to overflow urination and urinary retention.

Cutaneous symptoms include distal anhidrosis of the feet, excessive sweating of the trunk and sometimes gustatory sweating, which manifests facially in relation to food intake. [40]

Diagnosis of Symmetric and Distal Polyneuropathy.

Physician-patient interaction remains the foundational basis for diagnosis. A thorough interrogation should be performed, followed by a complete physical examination; on the other hand, non-invasive functional studies of diabetic patients with suspected neuropathy should be requested in case of diagnostic doubts and guided by the patient's clinical picture. [43]

All patients with type 2 Diabetes Mellitus should be screened at the time of diagnosis of diabetes and those with type 1 Diabetes Mellitus within five years of diagnosis, thereafter in both types at least once a year. Screening should include a careful history and physical examination that explores temperature or pinprick sensation (small fibre) and vibration sensation (large fibre). [49,50]

The diagnosis is basically clinical. There is no need for electrophysiological studies by electromyography and/or nerve conduction velocity when the history and physical findings are consistent with a diagnosis of diabetic neuropathy.

The test with the greatest relevance in clinical practice is the Michigan Neuropathy Screening Instrument (MNSI). This instrument was designed for outpatient use in primary care and is considered the standard for screening for diabetic neuropathy. This test has been reported to have a specificity of 95-100% and sensitivity of 57-93%. [50]

Another example of such a test is the Neuropathic Dysfunction Score (NDS), which examines cranial nerves, muscle weakness, reflexes and sensation. The scale consists of 35 items to compare between the left and right side of the body. This test is underused because it requires more training of the personnel performing the test.

The Neuropathy Impairment Score in the Lower Limbs (NIS-LLs) is a modified version of the NDS. It shows the degree of diabetic neuropathy impairment in the lower limbs, measures nerve function, pain and risk of foot ulceration and provides the best opportunity to assess therapeutic efficacy. [50,51]

Among the psychophysical methods, Quantitative Sensory Testing (QST), which allows the detection of early alterations in vibratory and thermal sensitivity and pain thresholds, requires special instruments and is not easily accessible in daily practice; it is recommended in case of suspected neuropathy in fine-calibre fibres. [51]

Nerve conduction studies are appropriate for the examination of long myelinated sensory and motor nerve fibres or in cases of advanced neuropathy. The limited availability of the necessary equipment and the costs involved mean that the clinical approach is given priority. [50]

The following clinical tests are used to assess the different nerve fibres:

1. Small fibre: prickling and temperature sensation.

2. Large fibres: vibration perception, proprioception, monofilament and ankle reflexes. [51]

To establish the diagnosis of diabetic polyneuropathy it is advised:
- Use simple scanning and tracking devices, cotton wool, pins, 128 Hz tuning fork and reflex hammer (examination of Achilles and patellar reflex), vibratory sensitivity in the first toe, assessment of tibialis anterior and peroneal muscle strength (heel and toe walking).

At least two out of three of the following pathological criteria should be present for the diagnosis of diabetic polyneuropathy:
- Typical symptoms such as burning, shooting pain, cramps, numbness, allodynia or hyperalgesia.
- Signs: decreased or abolished distal tactile sensitivity thresholds, impaired vibratory sensitivity, or distal tendon reflexes in a symmetrical manner; impaired thermal, vibratory (tuning fork) and pain sensitivity in a symmetrical manner. Symmetrical distal and symmetrical decreased and/or absent muscle strength (usually of late presentation).
- Alterations in electrophysiological studies (useful when objective figures are needed to assess nerve conduction velocities, both sensory and motor, latencies and amplitudes of the nerves studied). [50,51]

It is necessary to reach a diagnosis of damage to any area of the nervous system in patients with diabetes as early as possible, as involvement with multiple clinical manifestations is evidence of advanced neuropathy. It is with this criterion of early intervention that techniques have been developed and perfected to evaluate the lesion of thin fibres in order to diagnose fine fibre neuropathy, such as peripheral nerve biopsy and skin biopsy that evaluate the density of fibres at the intraepidermal level, as well as other histopathological characteristics that allow a diagnosis with a greater degree of certainty. [18]

It is essential to consider the multiple differential diagnoses that arise with other neuropathic disorders that may occur in a person with Diabetes Mellitus, such as endocrine-metabolic pathologies (uremic, amyloidosis, hypothyroidism), infectious (herpes, tabes, leprosy, HIV), nutritional (B-complex deficiency, alcoholism), hereditary: Pierre Marie Thot syndrome, toxic, by drugs: isoniazid, hydralazine, nitrofurantoin, disulfiram, vincristine, by metals (lead, gold); also inflammatory causes (paraneoplastic syndromes, rheumatological pathologies). [17,18]

Diagnosis of Diabetic Autonomic Neuropathy.

Screening for autonomic disease should be included in any evaluation of patients with diabetes mellitus. As the Autonomic Nervous System (ANS) is composed of small diameter and amyelinic fibres, its involvement is early in the progression of the disease,[38] being susceptible to metabolic noxa and subsequent hyperglycaemia-related pathways. It should therefore be noted that diabetic autonomic neuropathy may be present simultaneously with diabetic peripheral polyneuropathy. Despite its association with an increased risk of cardiovascular mortality and its association with impaired quality of life, the significance of autonomic neuropathy has not been fully appreciated. The reported prevalence varies widely according to the cohort studied and methods of assessment (9).

<u>Cardiac autonomic neuropathy.</u>

Tests that assess cardiovascular reflexes are the gold standard in the clinical diagnosis of cardiac dysautonomia. These tests have good sensitivity, specificity and reproducibility and are non-invasive, safe, standardised and relatively simple to perform. [9]

The first recommended clinical manoeuvre is the measurement of the heart rate; it should be assessed after the patient has been at rest for 5 to 10 minutes; a value equal to or greater than 90 beats per minute is a sign of tachycardia and may indicate the presence of vagal involvement; other causes (hyperthyroidism, fever) should always be ruled out. It is recommended to perform the following tests autonomic signs of vagal sympathetic involvement if the necessary tools are available. These tests allow investigation of heart rate variability in response to different stimuli such as change of decubitus, Valsalva manoeuvre and deep breathing. [40]

The analysis of the R-R spaces of the electrocardiogram during these tests allows to obtain the results that mark the normality or abnormality of the tests. Of these tests, heart rate variation with deep breathing has the highest specificity (around 80%). Sympathetic damage can be assessed by looking for orthostatic hypotension and performing the "hand-grip" manoeuvre or manual squeeze of a calibrated dynamometer or spring for 2 minutes. [50]

Confounding variables such as medications, hydration status and hypoglycaemia should be taken into account when performing these studies. People with diabetes mellitus who present with signs or symptoms of autonomic dysfunction such as unexplained tachycardia, orthostatic hypotension, poor exercise tolerance, should be evaluated for cardiac autonomic neuropathy. It is advisable to look for cardiac dysfunction from the diagnosis of type 2 diabetes mellitus and after 5 years of evolution in type 1 diabetes mellitus, especially in those at high risk for this complication due to poor chronic glycaemic control, cardiovascular risk factors, presence of somatic polyneuropathy and macro- and microangiopathic complications [51].

It is also advisable to measure the QT segment; there is evidence of a relationship between sudden death and QT segment length; this segment is an indicator of cardiac repolarisation and its regulation depends on the sympathetic nervous system; the normal QT value is < 440 milliseconds. [40] There are no systematised and standardised diagnostic criteria, so the staging of cardiac autonomic neuropathy is still a matter of debate. It is proposed that the presence of a cardiovagal test would identify the presence of possible or early involvement and it is proposed that at least 2 tests must be abnormal to confirm the diagnosis. The existence of orthostatic hypotension (asymptomatic or symptomatic) together with abnormal heart rate variability tests point to a severe or advanced condition of cardiac autonomic involvement. [51]

<u>Digestive tract neuropathy.</u>

It is important to clarify that symptomatology can be sparse and often non-specific, highly variable and, for reasons that are unclear, intermittent. [40-43]

The diagnosis of digestive tract involvement should be aimed at demonstrating the motility alterations that characterise it, bearing in mind that there are other pathologies with similar symptoms, which should be ruled out. In the interrogation, questions should be asked about the presence of postprandial fullness, constipation or diarrhoea. A very indicative sign is hypoglycaemia unrelated to mealtimes. [51]

At the oesophageal level, contrasted radiographic study may show mild dilatation, reduced primary peristaltic waves and prolonged transit. Intraluminal manometry is more sensitive. Neuropathological studies of the oesophagus have shown degenerative changes in the nerve trunks of the oesophageal plexus and in the proximity of the celiac ganglia. [14]

Methods used for the diagnosis of gastroparesis include: serial oesophagogastroduodenal radiography with barium meal, manometry, upper gastrointestinal endoscopy; scintigraphy (the gold standard) is performed using radioisotope-labelled solid and liquid food with gamma camera scans. The mean emptying time of liquids can be detected and should normally not exceed 10 minutes; that of solids is usually slower and should not exceed 100 minutes. The standardisation of the test meal has been improved, consisting of a low-fat intake, labelled with technetium 99.

The exhaled breath test using 13 C-acetate or octanoic acid is an interesting option, at least as a screening tool. Ultrasonography (two- or three-dimensional) is a non-invasive study and two-dimensional ultrasonography has been validated for the measurement of fluid and semi-solid emptying. Obesity, and the presence of gas in the bowel, in addition to the need for an experienced operator, limit the application of its use. The diagnosis of neurogenic diarrhoea is often reached by exclusion of other pathologies such as celiac disease, exocrine pancreatic insufficiency or bacterial superinfection. Simple radiology is non-specific and contrasted studies show prolonged transit with variations in the intestinal lumen, with dilated segments and thickening of the intestinal mucosa. [40,41]

<u>Genitourinary neuropathy.</u>

The first manoeuvre recommended for patients suspected of having a neurogenic bladder is to quantify the volume of the first morning micturition: figures greater than 400 ml suggest the presence of this disorder and justify complementary studies; the most commonly used is bladder ultrasound with measurement of postvoid residue; cystotonometry allows measurement of intravesical and intraurethral pressures. [51]

Urinary flowmetry and measurement of urethral nerve and sphincter potentials complete the diagnosis. Since they share the same autonomic innervation, the presence of neurogenic bladder is usually accompanied by sexual dysfunction, so it is essential to ask about it.

Diagnostic procedures for erectile dysfunction include the patient's medical and surgical history, questioning about the use of drugs with sexual impact, alcohol, tobacco and psychological aspects. Validated questionnaires such as the "Erectile Function Index" can be used to characterise the frequency and severity of symptoms. The nocturnal penile tumescence test, Doppler ultrasound of the penile vessels, bulbo cavernous reflexes, sensory conduction velocity studies, with measurement of the latency and amplitude of the dorsal penile nerves, and somatosensory evoked potentials of the pudendal nerves are other useful diagnostic measures. [11,22]

All these studies may be useful especially in patients who do not respond to 5-phosphodiesterase inhibitors. Injections of vasoactive substances such as phentolamine and papaverine can be used to check whether the involvement is predominantly vascular. Another aspect to consider is retrograde ejaculation associated with erectile dysfunction: this affects more than 35% of men with diabetes mellitus and is associated with sensory and autonomic neuropathy. To date, autonomic neuropathy has been considered the major organic component in the sexual dysfunction caused by Diabetes Mellitus [22].

Female sexual dysfunction is not systematically studied, but it is logical to infer its presence in women with neurogenic bladder and other stigmata of autonomic neuropathy; it is useful to ask about dyspareunia, especially in premenopausal women. [35,36]

The diagnosis of diabetic neuropathies is still fundamentally clinical, with valuable support from neurophysiological studies, especially neuroconduction and electromyography, which are vital in the differential diagnosis and characterisation of neuropathies. The most frequent diabetic neuropathies are distal sensory polyneuropathy and autonomic neuropathy. In addition to the duration and severity of diabetes, there are other independent risk factors in the genesis of neuropathy, such as lipid disorders, obesity and arterial hypertension. The presence of autonomic neuropathy, in addition to the clinical impact on the different systemic functions, in the case of cardiovascular involvement leads to higher mortality and lower life expectancy. [51]

Treatment of diabetic neuropathy.

Once the diagnosis of diabetic polyneuropathy has been made, intensive intervention is necessary to try to modify the progressive history of this microvascular complication. The first step is to optimise glycaemic control (aiming for HbA1c values below 7% as far as possible, but avoiding hypoglycaemias). [52]

<u>Treatment of painful neuropathy.</u>

Pain is one of the most disturbing manifestations of diabetic polyneuropathy; its treatment is often difficult and the patient should know that often only pain reduction will be achieved; nowadays there is a wide range of drugs that offer some degree of relief. The first conduct that should be established when faced with a patient with Diabetes Mellitus with neuropathic pain is that the diagnosis corresponds to a sensory affectation caused by diabetes, to differentiate it from other aetiologies of neuropathic pain (radicular compression, narrow spinal canal, traumatic affectation, etc.) that justify the symptom(s). [40]

It is clear that a favourable response is more likely in patients in whom early diagnosis is established, blood glucose is effectively reduced, measures are taken to avoid or reduce foot trauma, and timely and effective treatment of foot infections or ulcerations is initiated early, before they become uncontrollable. Weak analgesics can be used for moderate pain, but are not useful for severe pain, and long-term use of non-steroidal anti-inflammatory drugs is not recommended because of potential nephrotoxicity. Current treatment recommendations for painful diabetic neuropathy are as follows: [52]

Table 1. Recommendations for treatment of Diabetic Neuropathy Painful. [52]

Treatment line	Pharmacological Group	Drug	Dose
			recommended
1ª line of treatment	-Tricyclic antidepressants (Secondary Amines) -Selective norepinephrine and serotonin reuptake inhibitors (SNRIs) Calcium α2τ -Channel blockers Lidocaine patch 5% -Lidocaine patch 5% -Lidocaine patch 5% -Lidocaine patch 5% - Lidocaine patch	Amitriptyline Nortriptyline Desimipramine Duloxetine Venlafaxine Gabapentin Pregabalin	25-150mg/24h 25-150mg/24h 25-150mg/24h 30mg/24h-60mg/12h 37.5-225mg/24h 300-800mg/24h 75-150mg/24h Place the patch on the affected area for 12 hours. The maximum dose is 3 patches/day.
2nd line of treatment	Minor opioids Major opioids	Tramadol Morphine Oxycodone Methadone Transdermal fentanyl Transdermal buprenorphine	50-400mg/24h 10-20mg/12h 5-10mg/12h 2-5mg/24h 12-25mcg/h 15.5-35mcg/h
3ª line of treatment	Anticonvulsants Norepinephrine and dopamine reuptake inhibitors NMDA antagonists Capsaicin Topical 0.075%.	Carbamazepine Oxcarbacepine Topiramate Valproic acid Lamotrigine Clonazepam Bupropion Dextromorphan Mamantine	200-600mg/24h 300-2400mg/24h 100-800mg/24h 250-2000mg/24h 25-200mg/24h 0.5-4mg/24h 120-270mg/24h 30mg/24h 3-4 applications/day

Table 2. Anticonvulsants of choice in the treatment of Neuropathy Diabetic. [52]

	Mechanism	Dose Initial	Maintenance Dose (mg/d)	Interval (h)
Carbamazepine	↓ Channels Na⁺	200	600-1600	6-8
Oxcarbacepine	↓ Channels of Na⁺ ↓ Channels of Ca⁺² ⅛ Glutamate ↑ GABA	300	900-2400	12
Gabapentin	Blocking Ca channels⁺² dependent Na channels⁺	300	900-3600	8
Pregabalin	Ca channel blocking⁺² dependent channels	75	450	12
Clonazepam	↑ GABA	0.5	2-6	8-12
Topiramate	↑ GABA ↓ Glutamate	25	200-400	

The most frequently used drugs are:

- Analgesics: should be used with caution in diabetic patients due to the numerous interactions they present, also taking into account potential hepatotoxicity and gastric lesions, as well as the risk of addiction when opioids are used. Nonsteroidal anti-inflammatory drugs (NSAIDs) should not be prescribed as they have no effect on neuropathic pain; they can potentially cause renal compromise. The use of paracetamol to which dextroproxyfen or codeine can be added when the patient is very symptomatic usually provides relief. [52,53]

- Tricyclic antidepressants: the depression component is often seen in patients with chronic pain; tricyclic antidepressants (amitriptyline, imipramine and nortriptyline) have demonstrated efficacy in the clinic. This beneficial effect is independent of their antidepressant action and may be due to inhibition of neuronal reuptake of noradrenaline and serotonin and/or a direct effect on opioid receptors. Because of their anticholinergic activity, adverse events such as dry mouth and urinary retention are not uncommon. Due to the prolongation of the Qt segment associated with these drugs, arrhythmias may occur, so it is advisable to look for cardiac dysautonomia before using them. Both venlafaxine and duloxetine (dual-acting antidepressants) have demonstrated beneficial effects in neuropathic pain. The latter drug was approved by the Food and Drug Administration (FDA) for the treatment of painful neuropathy; it produces selective inhibition of noradrenaline and serotonin reuptake and maintains these neurotransmitters in the intersynaptic space. The most commonly used in Spain is amitriptyline, which has demonstrated efficacy for this indication. [52]

-   Anticonvulsants: Nerve hyperexcitability in pain transmission fibres is the main cause of neuropathic pain; in addition, spontaneous activity of primary afferent neurons in the dorsal horn of patients with peripheral neuropathy has been demonstrated. Glutamate, which acts on NMDA receptors, seems to play an important role in both mechanisms. All drugs that act by decreasing this nervous hyperexcitability or by decreasing glutamate levels will be effective in neuropathic pain. They are particularly useful when the pain is in the form of shooting crises, while they should be reserved if the pain is continuous. Occasionally, it may be necessary to combine more than one anticonvulsant to control pain and it should be noted that their onset of action does not begin before 3-4 weeks. Carbamazepine and deoxcarbazepine, at doses of 200-600 mg/day, have shown therapeutic efficacy. Gabapentin in doses of 400 mg to 3 g/day is another drug indicated for diabetic polyneuropathy pain; the most commonly reported side effects are dizziness and drowsiness. Currently, pregabalin (a chemical analogue of GABA that is inactive at GABA receptors) is the FDA-approved drug for the treatment of neuropathic pain. It is a ligand of the $\alpha 2\delta$ subunit of voltage-dependent calcium channels; beneficial effects in neuropathic pain are seen at doses of 300-600 mg/d. Somnolence, oedema and increased$_{peso.}$ are mentioned as the most frequent adverse events (53,54).

-   Local anaesthetics: act by blocking nerve conduction in altered afferent axons and decreasing the release of noradrenaline in sympathetic fibres. They are contraindicated in atrioventricular conduction disorders, heart failure and hepatic and renal failure. Lidocaine is administered in an initial dose of 1 mg/kg body weight dissolved in 250 ml of physiological saline to be given over 2 h. At weekly intervals, the infusion is repeated, increasing the dose up to 5 mg/kg lidocaine. Four to eight intravenous treatments are given. [54]

-   Opioids: although until a few years ago they were considered contraindicated in neuropathic pain, this is no longer the case and, although neuropathic pain responds less well to opioids than nociceptive pain, their use is becoming increasingly common in these patients. As in other types of chronic non-cancer pain, the use of potent opioids should be restricted to those patients with severe pain who do not respond to all other appropriate treatments. The opioid of choice is tramadol, because it has two mechanisms of action, binding to M opioid receptors and inhibition of noradrenaline and serotonin reuptake, the latter being the more potent effect. The usual dose is 50 mg every 8-6 h, with a maximum dose of 400 mg/day. If a potent opioid has to be administered, oxycodone can be used, which has good results in the treatment of neuropathic pain; it is recommended to start doses of 510 mg/12 h. Morphine sulphate can also be used due to its multiple presentations, which facilitate the titration of the patient's dose, transdermal fentanyl at a dose of 12 mg/h, transdermal buprenorphine 17.5-35 mg/h, and methadone due to its NMDA antagonist action. [54,55]

-   Topical preparations are used as a complementary treatment for elderly patients or those who cannot tolerate effective doses of analgesic drugs. As a topical drug, capsaicin, a substance contained in several species of capsicum peppers, has been approved for neuropathic pain: at high concentrations (8%), patching produces desensitisation to thermal and chemical noxae and mechanical stimuli in a dose-dependent fashion. [39] It is more effective in patients presenting superficial burning sensation than in those reporting deeper pain. May cause burning sensation, sneezing and coughing, rash and erythema as side effects. It should be applied three to four times a day in small amounts to avoid the unpleasant initial burning sensation, which disappears with successive applications. [52]

- Non-pharmacological approaches to pain such as transcutaneous, or percutaneous, nerve stimulation, application of frequency modulated electromagnetic waves, lasers and acupuncture are mentioned. The mode of action of these interventions is likely to be related to the release of endogenous opioids at the spinal cord level. The reported results are variable, but can be considered within the overall context of the indications. With regard to currently available drugs, one of them is thioctic acid, also known as alpha lipoic acid; this amphibolic substance, initially classified as a vitamin and synthesised in humans mainly in liver and kidney in trace amounts, has been attributed four main antioxidant properties and is therefore used in the treatment of diabetic neuropathy:

1. Ability to reduce reactive oxygen-derived species.
2. Ability to regenerate endogenous antioxidants.
3. Ability to repair oxidative tissue damage.
4. Chelating capacity.

It should be noted that drug combinations are usually necessary. A rational drug combination should be implemented with the aim of reducing pain and at the same time avoiding side effects with higher doses of a single drug, as they are usually dose-dependent. [40,52]

Treatment of autonomic neuropathy.

The most common symptomatic forms of diabetic autonomic neuropathy are gastroparesis, orthostatic hypotension and neurogenic bladder. [40]

Gastric motility disorders.

The aim of treatment is to increase the rate of evacuation of the stomach. Metoclopramide and domperidone have been shown to be useful, although their efficacy decreases with time of use and the extrapyramidal effects of the former drug should be mentioned given its ability to cross the blood-brain barrier. Cinitapride can also be used. Erythromycin, being a motilin receptor agonist, promotes gastric emptying. In situations of advanced involvement, it is indicated parenterally in the hospitalised patient. Synthetic motilin analogues are mentioned in the research stage, but there is still a lack of sustainable evidence. [40,42,43]

Treatment of orthostatic hypotension.

Often the use of therapeutic measures is unnecessary because the symptomatology is scarce and does not pose problems in the daily life of the patients. In those where symptoms are present (and in extreme cases may cause lipothymia), mechanical measures or the use of vasoconstrictive drugs are indicated. The former consist of raising the head of the bed by 10 to 12 cm, thereby reducing the pressure on the renal artery and promoting an increase in renin excretion with an increase in blood volume. Abrupt changes of position should be avoided. Another useful measure is the use of elastic bandages on the lower limbs or girdles that cover up to the costal area. This reduces the expansion capacity of the vascular bed when the postural change occurs. From the point of view of pharmacological indications, psychotropic drugs and diuretics should be eliminated in the first place. Treatment can be started with ephedrine in doses of 25-50 mg two to three times daily. If not successful, the use of glucocorticoids (fludrocortisone in initial doses of 1 mg for a few days, followed by maintenance treatment with 0.2 mg/d) improves hypotension. Midodrine can also be used in doses of 2.5 mg to 5 mg up to twice a day, which increases blood pressure and vascular tone, taking into account the side effects of alpha 1 adrenergic receptor agonism. [40,42]

<u>Neurogenic bladder.</u>

Treatment of neurogenic bladder is aimed at improving the dynamics of bladder emptying to avoid the postvoid residual urine that favours superimposed infections. In some cases the patient may self-catheterise and then be instructed to achieve voiding re-education, urinating on a scheduled basis, rather than waiting for the conscious sensation of bladder distension. Compression of the bladder through the abdominal wall may help to decrease voiding, but the possibility of increasing reflux to the kidneys should be remembered. Cholinergic agents such as bethanechol may facilitate bladder emptying, but there have been few controlled studies confirming their efficacy. Relaxation of the internal sphincter of the bladder neck can be achieved with alpha-blockers such as doxazosin at 1 or 2 mg, two to three times daily. [40]

The existing clinical and epidemiological evidence affirms the high prevalence of diabetic neuropathy; it is the earliest and most frequent of the microvascular complications. Hence the need for early diagnosis in the diabetic population to avoid the high personal, family and occupational costs of this compromise. The main objective is prevention, for which it is necessary to ensure that both the healthcare team and patients receive the necessary education to avoid neuropathy and, once it has developed, to slow its progression. It should be borne in mind that the involvement of the entire nervous system and not just the limbs. Within the involvement of the ANS, the wide field of dysautonomia can have a profound impact on quality of life and also on life expectancy. If neuropathy has not been prevented, appropriate pharmacological, aetiopathogenic and symptomatic measures should be implemented in order to slow down its progression. [44]

III. Integral Care Programme for Diabetic Patients.

For more than 40 years, the National Institute of Endocrinology in Cuba has designed the National Programme of Comprehensive Care for Diabetic Patients with the aim of reducing morbidity and mortality in patients with diabetes mellitus; this programme has been modified over the years, adapting to the social and economic changes in the country.

Optimal diabetes care by health care providers and patients can prevent or delay the development of complications, hence a well-designed comprehensive diabetes care programme can lead to significant reductions in morbidity, disability and premature mortality.

This programme does not operate in isolation, its actions are enhanced by training, integration of services at all levels of the Health System, especially in close interaction with other programmes for the prevention and treatment of Chronic Non-Communicable Diseases. [23]

Most diabetic patients are cared for in the primary care units/family doctor system (where adequate training needs to be ensured as the component of the system closest to the patient), with adequate integration of the referral and counter-referral system with the secondary and tertiary levels.

Among the objectives of the programme are to improve knowledge of the magnitude of the diabetes mellitus problem in Cuba and to support research aimed at the prevention and control of this disease. To this end, training of health care providers, patients and their families at all levels of the system is of paramount importance. [23]

The Cuban programme for diabetic patients refers to the search for risk factors and symptoms associated with vegetative or autonomic neuropathic disorders from the first consultation, as well as the appropriate and exhaustive neurological physical examination. On the other hand, it establishes that after the initial comprehensive assessment, the patient must be seen in consultation and field at least every four months and a complete neurological assessment annually. A complete physical examination, with special reference to weight, blood pressure, cardiovascular, neurological and lower limb examinations, should be carried out at quarterly consultations. A metabolic control record should also be established, including the patient's own blood glucose check four times a day (before breakfast, lunch, dinner and at bedtime), all of which should be recorded in the medical record, as well as a lipid profile every six months.

Although the programme recognises diabetic neuropathy as a highly prevalent complication in the diabetic population, there is no exhaustive reference to its forms of presentation or behaviour to be taken into account in patients who present with it, with the exception of the diabetic foot as the final stage of the neuropathic complication in the lower limbs, i.e. there is no evidence of equal interest and knowledge of it compared to other complications of diabetes mellitus, which leads to its late detection.

The wide universe of this complication makes it necessary for the medical professional who cares for people with diabetes to have an open and integrated view of it. On the other hand, ignorance of this condition leads to a decrease in its detection, which increases morbidity and mortality in patients with diabetes mellitus. It is clear that the management and treatment of this chronic complication of diabetes mellitus is a significant challenge that requires knowledge and preparation on the part of the primary health care physician. [20]

4 METHODOLOGICAL DESIGN

Research was carried out on health systems and services through a descriptive observational study in the health area of the "Manuel Piti Fajardo" Teaching Polyclinic in Santo Domingo, in the period from September/2021 to June/2023.

Sample.

Two samples were selected for the study, one of patients and the other of health professionals.

<u>Patients:</u>

The study consisted of 54 diabetic patients over 40 years of age, with a diagnosis of diabetic neuropathy for more than one year, who attended the Comprehensive Care Consultation for Diabetic Patients at the "Manuel Piti Fajardo" polyclinic during the period from September/2021 to June/2023.

For inclusion in the study, patients expressed their willingness to participate by signing the informed consent form (Appendix 1).

<u>Health professionals:</u>

We worked with 35 doctors in the health area of Santo Domingo, selected by means of a non-probabilistic purposive sample. All the Residents of 1er, 2do and 3er year and the Specialists in General Comprehensive Medicine belonging to the two Basic Work Groups (GBT) of the urban area, who were providing care in the study period and who gave their consent to participate in the study, were included (Annex 1A). (Annex 1A).

The study consisted of the tactical evaluation of some elements corresponding to the structure and process components of the Integrated Diabetic Patient Care Programme related to diabetic neuropathy.

In the **structure component**, staff qualifications, competence and experience were analysed, and in the **process component**, the quality of care (diagnostic and therapeutic) was analysed, specifically with regard to the early detection and timely treatment of diabetic neuropathy.

Data collection methods and techniques.

In the first stage, a detailed interrogation was carried out using an Individual Interview Guide (Annex 2) prepared after a review of the updated bibliography, which consisted of two parts.

The first part collected general data on the patient and data of interest for the research, which referred to the characterisation of the study group and included the variables age, sex, skin colour, smoking habits and alcoholic beverage intake.

The second part of this instrument was applied to the patients in order to identify the neuropathic symptoms and signs and the time of their evolution. It consisted of 30 questions related to the different types of neuropathy, which were written in a simple way, avoiding the use of medical terminology, in order to achieve a better understanding by the patients in the study.

To complete the collection of information, a physical examination was carried out to look for the presence in the patients of symptoms and signs of diabetic neuropathy; this included the determination of blood pressure; the calculation of the body mass index; the search for foot deformities and special emphasis was placed on the neurological examination, determining the patients' pain and vibration sensitivity, as well as the osteotendinous reflexes. This physical examination was carried out by the researcher together with the doctor from the "Manuel Piti Fajardo" Polyclinic's Diabetic Patient Comprehensive Care Clinic.

-A sphygmomanometer certified as suitable for use by the Department of Metrology and Standardisation was used to measure blood pressure, and the procedure was carried out on the left upper limb with the patient in a sitting position. A 15-minute rest period was taken into account before taking the blood pressure and some factors that could modify the results of the test were ruled out beforehand, such as physical exercise prior to taking the blood pressure, drinking coffee or other stimulants, and smoking 30 minutes before taking the blood pressure.

- On the other hand, the calculation of the body mass index (BMI) included the determination of body weight and height, for which the scale of the Diabetic Comprehensive Care Clinic was used, which was certified as suitable for use by the Department of Metrology and Standardisation, while for the determination of height, the measuring rod attached to the scale was used.

- The neurological examination was performed in a calm and relaxed environment. For the exploration of painful and vibratory sensitivity, a hypodermic needle and a 128 Hz tuning fork were used respectively, for which the patient was placed in supine decubitus with eyes closed to avoid falsifying the results, and so that the patient would not memorise the exploratory sequence, this was carried out randomly without following a pre-established order.

In the case of vibratory sensitivity, a 128 Hz tuning fork was held at the base and a sharp blow was applied to produce vibration, and then placed perpendicularly on a bony prominence with constant pressure. Sensitivity was explored at the level of both malleoli and at the level of the distal phalanx of the first toe of both feet.

For pain sensitivity, a hypodermic needle was used for each patient, applying a painful stimulus, with special emphasis on the plantar region of both lower limbs and the plantar area of the first and fifth metatarsal.

The patient indicated in each case with an affirmative (Yes) or negative (No) response in correspondence with the perception or not of the stimulus respectively. The examination was avoided in areas where there were ulcers, wounds or other dermatological lesions.

-To explore the osteotendinous or deep reflexes, we took as a reference the Achilles or triceps sural reflex, with the subject kneeling on a chair or stretcher, the explorer lifted the patient's foot slightly with one hand and with the other hand the reflex hammer was tapped at the level of the Achilles tendon, taking care not to tap the calcaneus. The patient's normal response should have been extension of the foot. It was considered altered when this response was not observed when this manoeuvre was performed.

- The complementary examination included the determination of total cholesterol and triglycerides, fasting and postprandial blood glucose, as well as the performance of an electrocardiogram.

The preparation for blood sampling was based on the following requirements: having eaten a light meal the night before, fasting for 12 to 14 hours, and not having drunk alcoholic beverages 24 hours before. A microcentrifuge (KOKUSAN) was used for the determinations, after coordination with the Clinical Laboratory located in the health area where the samples were taken for the research, which was in accordance with the quality standards for this purpose and was certified as suitable for use by the Department of Metrology and Standardisation.

-Each patient underwent an electrocardiogram to determine the heart rate at rest, as well as any other alterations that the patient might present, for which purpose the patient removed all metallic objects he or she possessed, such as belts, watches, rings, earrings, etc. Once the patient was barefoot and in the supine decubitus position on the stretcher, the area of the thorax where the electrodes were placed was cleaned with a cotton wool soaked in alcohol for the subsequent electrocardiogram.

The data were completed by reviewing the individual medical records of the patients in the sample, using a Documentary Review Guide (Annex 3), which helped to determine whether or not a timely diagnosis of diabetic neuropathy was made and whether the medical follow-up was carried out with the quality and frequency of consultations and interconsultations established by the programme. In addition, important data were obtained such as the type of diabetes mellitus and the time of its evolution, associated comorbidities, the treatment indicated, the frequency of consultations received by the patient in the last five years and the quality of these consultations.

In addition, a questionnaire was applied to Primary Care doctors (Annex 4) designed by the research team following the experience of previous research. In order to carry out the questionnaire, the updated bibliography was consulted and a round table discussion was held with the research team where the five thematic nuclei to be evaluated were defined (Generalities of Diabetic Neuropathy, Clinical Manifestations of Diabetic Neuropathy, Affectation by systems of Diabetic Neuropathy, Diagnosis and Treatment of Diabetic Neuropathy); this questionnaire was made up of two sections. The first of these was designed with the purpose of collecting general data of interest for the research, such as degree of specialisation, participation in postgraduate courses received in the last five years on the subject of diabetic neuropathy and knowledge of an instrument or tool used to evaluate the presence of diabetic neuropathy. The second part of this instrument allowed us to determine the level of knowledge that the health professionals possessed about diabetic neuropathy, which was evaluated in correspondence with what was established in the qualification key (Annex 5).

Operationalisation of variables.

In the patient sample:

<u>Epidemiological and clinical variables of interest.</u>

1. Age: years of age at the time of the research. The following age groups were

defined:

- Between 40 and 49 years old.
- Between 50 and 59 years old.
- Between 60 and 69 years old.
- Over 70 years old.

2. Sex: according to biological sex.

-Female (F).

-Male (M).

3. Skin colour: according to skin colour.

- White (B).
- Non White (NB).

4. Smoking habit: taking into account the information obtained from the Individual Interview Guide (Annex 2), the following categories were established: -Active smoker.

-Passive smoking.

Ex-smoker.

-No Smoking.

5. Consumption of alcoholic beverages: taking into account the information obtained from the Individual Interview Guide (Annex 2), the following categories were established:

-Yes: when the patient has a history of drinking alcoholic beverages regardless of the type, quantity and frequency of consumption.

-No: when the patient had no history of drinking alcoholic beverages.

6. Type of Diabetes Mellitus: endocrine metabolic disorder, due to alterations in the metabolism of carbohydrates, fats and proteins, due to a relative or absolute deficit in the synthesis of insulin or a defect in the use of insulin. Taking into account the information obtained from the Documentary Review Guide (Annex 3), the following were defined:

- Diabetes Mellitus type 1.
- Diabetes Mellitus type 2.

7. Time course of diabetes mellitus: period of time from diagnosis of the disease to the time of the investigation:

- Under 5 years old.
- Between 5 and 10 years.
- Between 10 and 15 years.
- More than 15 years.

8. Comorbidities present in the patient: taking into account the information obtained from the Documentary Review Guide (Annex 3):

- Arterial Hypertension.
- Chronic Kidney Disease.
- Ischaemic heart disease.
- Dyslipidaemia.

-    Obesity.

9.   Degree of metabolic control: prognostic assessment of the patient's metabolic control based on clinical and biochemical parameters.

<u>Clinical parameters:</u>

- Presence or absence of symptoms.

1) Nothing to report-Well.

2) Polyuria, polyphagia, polydipsia, asthenia, paraesthesia, weight loss - Bad.

- Nutritional assessment: this was carried out by determining the Body Mass Index (BMI).

1)   18,5-24,9 Kg/m^2 Normopeso.

2)   25-29.9 Kg/m^2 Overweight.

3)   >30- Kg/m^2 Obese.

It was interpreted as set out below:

1)   Normo peso- Good.

2)   Overweight - Acceptable.

3)   Obese - Bad.

- Blood pressure

1) < 130/85 mmHg - Good.

2) >130/85 mmHg - <140/90 mmHg - Acceptable.

3)>140-90 mmHg - Bad.

<u>Biochemical parameters:</u>

- Fasting Blood Glucose Levels.

1)   < 6.1 mmol/l- Good.

2)6.1 - 7 mmol/l- Acceptable.

3)>7 mmol/l- Bad.

- Postprandial Blood Glucose Levels.

1) < 7.8 mmol/l- Good.

2)7.8 -10 mmol/l- Acceptable.

3)>10 mmol/l- Bad.

Lipid levels.

- Total Cholesterol.

1) < 5.2 mmol/l- Good.

2)5,2 - 6,2 mmol/l- Acceptable.

3)> 6.2 mmol/l- Bad.

- Triglycerides.

1)   < 1.7 mmol/l- Good.

2)1.7 - 2.2 mmol/l- Acceptable.

3)> 2.2 mmol/l- Bad.

For the distribution of the degree of metabolic control of the patients, the variables were interpreted as follows:

1)   Good metabolic control: when all clinical and biochemical parameters were classified as good.

2) Acceptable metabolic control: when all parameters were in the acceptable category or when combinations of the seven parameters alternated between acceptable and good in any of their variants.

3) Poor metabolic control: when there were one or more poor criteria and the others were in the good or acceptable category.

10. Type of Diabetic Neuropathy: a microvascular complication characterised by signs or symptoms of peripheral nerve dysfunction affecting the somatic and autonomic system in patients with Diabetes Mellitus type 1 and 2.

-Symmetrical and distal polyneuropathy: when the patient was found on physical examination to have sensory-motor involvement, predominantly in the lower limbs, with insidious and centripetal progression, with predominance of sensory symptoms, either by excess: paraesthesia, allodynia, and reporting nocturnal pain that improves with walking (small fibre involvement) or by default: hypoesthesia, ataxia, areflexia (coarse fibre involvement); and when affirmative answers were obtained to the questions from items 1 to 13 in the second part of the Individual Patient Interview Guide. (Annex 2)

- Autonomic or vegetative neuropathy: involvement of both the sympathetic and parasympathetic systems, in a patchy manner, associated with various clinical symptoms, depending on the territory affected.

• Gastrointestinal: when the patient presented a history of gastroparesis, diarrhoea predominantly at night, constipation, faecal incontinence, nausea, vomiting, early satiety with colicky abdominal pain and hypoglycaemia not related to meal times, and also took into account the affirmative answers from items 16-21 obtained from the second part of the Individual Patient Interview Guide (Annex 2).

• Genitourinary: when the patient presented a history of neurogenic bladder, severe urinary incontinence, erectile dysfunction, retrograde ejaculation and dyspareunia, in addition, the affirmative answers from items 22 to 27 obtained from the second part of the Individual Patient Interview Guide were taken into account (Annex 2).

• Cardiovascular: when the patient was found to have sinus tachycardia, prolongation of the QT interval, decreased R-R variability, orthostatic hypotension and poor exercise tolerance, and the affirmative answers to the questions from items 28 to 30 in the second part of the Individual Patient Interview Guide were also taken into account (Annex 2).

-Mixed: when the patient presented with autonomic system involvement (cardiovascular, gastrointestinal and genitourinary) as well as clinical manifestations of symmetrical and distal polyneuropathy.

<u>Variables to determine quality in the follow-up and control of diabetic patients.</u>

11. Quality in monitoring and control.

It was determined from the review of individual clinical histories and taking into account the follow-up and control of diabetic patients in the last five years of evolution of the disease; taking the following criteria, indicators and standards as a reference:

Criteria	Indicators	Standard

		r
Frequency of Consultations and Grounds.	Number of patients with adequate consultation frequency / *Total patients* × 100	100
Anamnesis .	Number of patients with correct anamnesis − × 100 / *Total patients*	100
Examination Physical.	Number of patients with complete physical examination and cori / *Total patients* × 100	100
Laboratory examinations.	Number of patients with established laboratory tests by programme indicated *Total patients* × IOO	100
	Number of patients with established laboratory tests per programme performed *Total number of patients* × 100	90
Diagnostic Impression.	Number of patients with a correct diagnosis *Total number of patients* × 100	90
Timely diagnosis of diabetic neuropathy	Number of patients with a timely diagnosis of diabetic neuropathy / *Total patients* × 100	90
Medical Indications.	Number of patients with appropriate medical indications × 100 / *Total patients*	100
Medical thinking or judgement about risk of diabetic neuropathy.	Number of patients with recommendations for modifying risk factors for dial neuropathy / *Total patients* × 100	'100

In such a way that:

J The frequency of consultations and diabetic patient plots was considered adequate when two consultations and one plot per year were recorded in the clinical history.

J An adequate anamnesis was considered adequate when the medical history included the personal and family pathological history, the general and device-related symptoms reported by the patient, the presence of symptoms related to the different forms of presentation of diabetic neuropathy and the time of evolution of these symptoms.

J A complete and correct physical examination was considered to have been carried out when it covered the general, regional and apparatus physical examination and when the four basic techniques were used during the clinical examination: inspection, palpation, auscultation and percussion in each of the systems in order to recognise the existence or not of physical alterations or signs of the disease; The sphygmomanometer was also used to measure blood pressure, and other devices such as the 128 Hz tuning fork and the hammer for neurological examination of the patient, with emphasis on superficial and deep sensitivity, osteotendinous reflexes, trophism of the lower limbs and the presence or absence of lesions, ulcers or deformities in the feet.

J The indicated laboratory tests were considered to be in line with the programme when they were indicated at least twice a year and included at least blood glucose, total cholesterol and triglycerides.

J A correct diagnosis of diabetic neuropathy was considered to be established when it was related to the information obtained from the anamnesis, the general, regional and apparatus physical examination, as well as the correct interpretation of the indicated laboratory tests.

J A timely diagnosis of diabetic neuropathy was considered to have been made when the time between the onset of symptoms and the initial diagnosis was less than 4 months.

J The medical indications were considered to be adequate when they corresponded to the established diagnosis and the type of neuropathy present in the patient, with special emphasis on the pharmacological and non-pharmacological treatment guidelines.

J Adequate medical judgement on the risk of diabetic neuropathy was considered to be established when recommendations for modification of the risk factors for neuropathy in each patient were recorded in the individual medical record.

<u>Variables referring to health professionals.</u>

12. Specialisation: according to the degree of specialisation attained by the doctor and the studies he/she is currently pursuing. Based on the information collected in the questionnaire (Annex 4), these were defined:

- R1: First Year Resident in General Comprehensive Medicine.
- R2: Second Year Resident in General Comprehensive Medicine.
- R3: Third Year Resident in General Comprehensive Medicine.
- E: Specialist in General Comprehensive Medicine.

13. Postgraduate courses received related to diabetic neuropathy: according to what the professional referred to in the questionnaire (Annex 4), two categories were established:

- Yes: when the professional reported having received one or more postgraduate courses on the subject in the last five years.
- No: otherwise.

14. Knowledge of an instrument or tool used to assess the presence of diabetic neuropathy: as reported by the practitioner in the questionnaire (Annex 4), two

categories were established:

-   Yes: when the practitioner correctly checked one or more tools to assess for the presence of diabetic neuropathy.
-   No: otherwise.

15. Knowledge needs: this referred to the knowledge demanded by the doctors about Diabetic Neuropathy when applying the questionnaire (Annex 4). For the quantitative evaluation of the questionnaire by thematic nuclei and in general, a rating key was used (Annex 5), where the following categories were defined:

Evaluation by thematic cores on the basis of 20 total points:

Low knowledge needs:	18 to 20 points.
Average knowledge needs:	14 to 17 points.
High knowledge needs:	Less than 14 points.

Overall assessment on the basis of 100 total points:

Low knowledge needs:	90 to 100 points.
Average knowledge needs:	70 to 89 points.
High knowledge needs	Less than 70 points.

ethical aspects.

The research team was responsible for explaining the objectives of the study to each of the participants. They were informed that the information collected was confidential and for scientific, research and training purposes without violating any of the established ethical principles, and that the information was archived to guarantee its security. Furthermore, it was made clear that the identity of each participant would be preserved and that the questionnaire to the professionals would be anonymous. The individual decision of the professionals not to cooperate with the research was respected, for which the model of informed consent (Annex 1A) was taken into account, and a request for authorisation was made to the management of the entity for the development of the research (Annex 1B).

Statistical analysis.

The data were stored in the general database system Microsoft Excel to facilitate their analysis. Subsequently, statistical processing was carried out using SPSS ("Statistical Package for Social Sciences") version 22 for Windows. The resulting information was presented in frequency tables where descriptive statistics such as absolute frequencies and percentages were used. The test of independence based on the Chi-square distribution was applied to evaluate the possible association between two qualitative variables. As a result, the value of its statistic (X^2) was shown, as well as the significance associated with it (p).

Hypothesis testing:

Ho: There is no association between the variables.

H1: There is an association between the variables.

Statistical significance was interpreted according to the following criteria:

- If $p > 0.05$ There is no significant association between the variables.
- If $p \leq 0.05$ there is a significant association between the variables.

A reliability level of 95% was set.

The results obtained from the statistical processing and synthesis were used to create tables and graphs for better analysis and understanding.

5 RESULTS

The distribution of patients according to age and type of neuropathy (Table 1), showed a predominance of symmetrical and distal polyneuropathy for 50.0%; mainly in the age range of 70 years and over with 25.9%. This was followed in frequency by mixed neuropathy with a total of 11 patients for 20.4%, the majority being patients over 70 years of age (11.1%). A lower prevalence of cardiovascular (12.9%), gastrointestinal (9.2%) and genitourinary (7.4%) autonomic neuropathy was observed.

In the distribution of the patients in the study group according to sex and skin colour (Table 2 and 3 respectively), a predominance of females was observed with a representation of 33 patients for 61.1%, of whom 31.5% presented symmetrical and distal neuropathy, this type of neuropathy being the most frequent in the female sex as well as in the male sex with 18.5% in relation to the total. In terms of skin colour, white patients accounted for 75.9%.

With regard to smoking (Table 4), it was found that all the forms of neuropathy included in the study were more frequent in active smokers (48.1%) than in non-smokers (16.6%). The number of ex-smoking patients who developed some form of neuropathy was also significant at 20.4% of the total (11 patients).

With regard to alcoholic beverage intake, 53.7% of the sample consumed alcoholic beverages, of which 16 developed distal symmetrical polyneuropathy for 29.6% of the total number of patients included in the study. However, it was evident that in the case of autonomic neuropathies (Cardiovascular 7.4%, Gastrointestinal and Genitourinary both with a representativeness of 3.7%) and mixed (11.1%) there was a predominance in patients with no history of alcoholic beverage consumption. (Table 5)

The distribution in terms of type of diabetes and type of neuropathy (Table 6) showed that patients with type 2 diabetes mellitus developed some form of this complication to a greater extent, accounting for 87.0% of all cases, with the number of patients with symmetrical and distal polyneuropathy standing out at 46.3%, followed in order of frequency by mixed neuropathy at 18.5% in this group of patients; In patients with type 1 diabetes mellitus, there were an equal number of patients with symmetrical and distal polyneuropathy and autonomic neuropathy of the cardiovascular type with two cases respectively, which constituted 3.7%.

Considering the evolution of diabetes mellitus (Table 7), the highest number of patients with some form of diabetic neuropathy was found in the range of 10-15 years of diabetes mellitus evolution with 40.7% (22 patients). This was followed by patients with an evolution of diabetes mellitus older than 15 years (27.8%) where the predominant type of neuropathy was symmetrical and distal polyneuropathy with nine patients (16.6%). In third place, patients with an evolution of their disease between 5 and 10 years (16.6%), and lastly, those with an evolution of less than five years (14.8%).

Table 8 summarised the distribution of patients according to comorbidities and type of neuropathy, which showed that 40.7% had arterial hypertension, followed by 11 patients with ischaemic heart disease, representing 20.4%, and 16.6% had dyslipidaemia.

When analysing metabolic control, we can conclude from the results of the research that the majority of patients who developed some form of neuropathy had poor metabolic control (40.7%), followed in order by those with acceptable control (35.1%). Patients with poor metabolic control presented mainly symmetrical and distal polyneuropathy with 20.4% (11 patients) as shown in table 9.

With regard to the adequate quality of follow-up and control of diabetic patients, it was found that none of the indicators analysed scored according to the pre-established standard, with the most critical scores being, in order, the timely diagnosis of diabetic neuropathy (33.0%), the frequency of consultations and medical grounds (46.2%), the establishment of a correct diagnostic impression in each case (49.1%) and the adequate physical examination of patients (51.0%), as shown in Table 10.

The distribution of health professionals according to degree of specialisation showed that, of the 35 doctors who participated in the research, ten (28.6%) were first-year residents, seven (20.0%) second-year residents, five (14.3%) third-year residents and thirteen specialists in General Comprehensive Medicine, the latter predominating with 37.1%, as shown in Graph 1.

100% of the professionals reported not having attended postgraduate courses related to the topic of Diabetic Neuropathy in the last five years and none of them were aware of the tools that can be used to assess the presence of this complication.

With regard to the final evaluation according to level of specialisation (Table 11), the results showed that, in general, healthcare personnel need to be informed about Diabetic Neuropathy. 65.7% of the professionals had a high need for knowledge about this neuropathic complication. Second year residents had the worst results, with 71.4% presenting a high need for knowledge, followed in order by first year residents with 70.0%, General Comprehensive Medicine specialists with 61.5% and finally third year residents with 60.0%. According to the statistical results, there is no significant association between knowledge and type of professional (p=0.9970), which reflects that there is a need for learning about this subject regardless of the doctors' degree of specialisation.

When analysing the degree of general knowledge by thematic area assessed by all the doctors who participated in the study (Table 12), it was found that the greatest difficulties were in knowledge of Diagnosis (77.1%). In the area of Generalities, 74.3% had a high expressed need for knowledge. Similarly, in the Affectation by Systems, although with a lower percentage (71.4%), it was found that the results achieved were unfavourable. With regard to Clinical Manifestations and Treatment, both with 62.9%, no satisfactory results were obtained either, although a greater number of professionals achieved better scores in this area than in the others. Hypothesis testing showed no significant differences between the knowledge needs of these professionals and the content addressed in each of the thematic areas of the questionnaire (p=0.8705), which is clear evidence that physicians are insufficiently prepared in all areas related to this complication of diabetes mellitus.

When addressing the knowledge needs of the specialists in General Comprehensive Medicine with regard to diabetic neuropathy (Table 13), by aspect evaluated, it was observed that in all aspects they obtained very unfavourable results. The greatest difficulties were related to the general aspects and the diagnosis of diabetic neuropathy, so that in both 76.9% presented a high need for information on this subject. In nine specialists (69.2%) there was a high need for knowledge on the Clinical Manifestations of Diabetic Neuropathy. There was also a deficient mastery of Systemic Affections and Treatment, both with 61.5%. The hypothesis test in this case showed that there were no significant differences (p=0.9599), thus demonstrating that there is a great lack of knowledge about this chronic complication of diabetes in these specialists regardless of the content addressed in each thematic nucleus in relation to diabetic neuropathy.

The knowledge needs of the First Year Residents, by aspect assessed, are shown in table 14. In eight of the ten first year residents, high knowledge needs related to the diagnosis were diagnosed. 70.0% also answered incorrectly on the general aspects of this complication, systemic involvement and treatment. While six had difficulties regarding the clinical manifestations that can occur in diabetic neuropathy. The hypothesis test showed no significant differences (p=0.7513), thus demonstrating that there is a poor mastery of the contents addressed in each of the thematic nuclei.

With regard to the knowledge needs of the Second Year Residents by aspect evaluated (Table 15), the worst results were related in equal measure to the Affectation by Systems and in the Diagnosis of Diabetic Neuropathy, both subjects with equal percentages (85.7%), followed by knowledge of the Generalities of this complication (71.4%). A poor command of Clinical Manifestations and Treatment was also found in four second-year residents (57.1%). The hypothesis test on these aspects showed that there were no significant differences (p=0.8867), thus demonstrating that there is a great lack of knowledge about diabetic neuropathy regardless of the sections evaluated in each thematic axis.

In relation to the Third Year Residents, we were able to confirm that the greatest difficulties were reflected in the thematic nuclei dealing with the generalities and affectation by systems in diabetic neuropathy in four of the five residents (80.0%). In the rest of the topics evaluated, no satisfactory results were obtained either, which showed high knowledge needs in three residents, in the aspects dealing with Clinical Manifestations, Diagnosis and Treatment for 60.0% each, as shown in Table 16. The hypothesis test on these aspects showed that there are no significant differences (p=0.8240) in relation to the theoretical hypothesis, thus demonstrating that there is a great lack of knowledge about diabetic neuropathy in this group of doctors and that the aspects dealt with in each thematic nucleus do not influence the results achieved by these professionals.

6 DISCUSSION

Diabetic neuropathy is a major global health problem and the number one complication of diabetes. Hence, improving the quality of care for diabetic patients at all levels represents both a challenge and an opportunity to reduce the direct and indirect costs of the disease and in turn improve the quality of life of patients. [56]

In the present study, a predominance of symmetrical and distal polyneuropathy was found, which was significantly higher in women compared to men, as well as an increase in neuropathy with age, with a higher frequency of this complication in patients aged 70 years and older. These results are in agreement with those reported by Dr. Vintimilla Molina and her collaborators[39] in an intervention carried out in Ecuador, where the frequency is also higher in women (49.3%), and also establishes that the increase in this complication is directly proportional to the age of the patients. We also agree with Dr. Flores-Cuevas[49] who supports the predominance of females with this complication and considers symmetrical and distal neuropathy as the main clinical form in relation to autonomic neuropathy which constitutes only 22.0% of the sample studied in this research. However, we disagree with Di Lorenzi[19] who states in his study that there are no differences between the sexes in the development of neuropathy as a complication of diabetes mellitus.

In relation to smoking, we agree with the results presented in other studies such as that of Dr. Chaviano Belette[18] and Di Lorenzi[19] who recognise toxic habits as highly important risk factors in the development of neuropathy, especially smoking, which is considered to have an oxidative effect on cells and nerve fibres, an essential pillar in the pathogenesis of this neuropathic complication.

With regard to the comorbidities that occurred most frequently in the patients in the study, our results are similar to those reported by Dr. Aguillón de Ramírez[57] in her article where she states that high blood pressure, dyslipidemias and obesity are the diseases most frequently suffered by the patients in the sample in her research.

Ramírez-López[20] points out the importance of screening and control of chronic diseases in diabetic patients, especially hypertension and dyslipidaemia, as these are risk factors involved in the onset of neuropathy.

Regarding the type of diabetes, patients with type 2 diabetes mellitus developed the highest prevalence of this complication. Similar results were found in the study by Di Lorenzi[19] in Uruguay, who reported a prevalence of neuropathy of 34.6%, which is more frequent in the population with type 2 diabetes mellitus. This is closely related to the longer evolution of the disease, as well as to advanced age and dyslipidaemia.

In our study, neuropathy predominated in patients with an evolution of diabetes of 10 to 15 years. The time of evolution is one of the most important factors for the development of diabetic neuropathy; in most of the literature, its presence has been reported in more than 10 years of diabetes evolution; however, in our research we conclude that with less than 10 years of diagnosis there are already signs of diabetic neuropathy. Furthermore, we can highlight that the highest number of patients with some variant of neuropathy were those with poor metabolic control. Our results correspond with the incidence reported by Dr. González García[55] in her research where more than half of the patients with diabetic neuropathy have poor metabolic control. Likewise, this coincides with the results of the analysis carried out by the European Diabetes Prospective Complications Study (EURODIAB)[51] in which it is established that the cumulative incidence of diabetic neuropathy is related to inadequate glycaemic control and the longer duration of Diabetes Mellitus. On the other hand, Dr. Vintimilla Molina[39] reports in her study that the frequency of peripheral neuropathy of the lower limbs increases with age (the longer the exposure to diabetes, the greater the probability of neuropathy).

Unfortunately, diabetic neuropathy is diagnosed in advanced stages, which is due to various factors, ranging from a limited time for medical consultation and also due to the lack of knowledge of professionals to make a timely diagnosis. Early diagnosis at the first level of care through screening can greatly reduce complications and the risk of disability and thus give the patient a better quality of life. For this reason, it is essential that the family doctor has the knowledge, skills and abilities to diagnose it. [58]

Internationally, there is growing recognition of the importance of evaluation of specific programmes as a measure of the efficacy, effectiveness, utility, efficiency and safety, as well as the cost-benefit of a new or improved health technology or service, and the implicit impact on the quality of services, satisfaction and well-being of increasingly informed users, who demand better outcomes. [59]

The evaluation will also serve to make decisions about the programme as it develops "feed back", as a quality control system vis-à-vis the user; in this case, the population group on which we are trying to have an impact, and it is a useful instrument that allows changes or adjustments in the implementation policies of the programmes. [59,60]

The evaluation of the process component in this study showed that none of the indicators analysed scored according to the pre-established standard. We found similar results in the study carried out in the "Hermanos Cruz" polyclinic in Havana where Dr. Casanova Moreno[61] , demonstrates that there are difficulties in complying with the diabetes education programme for older adults in the health area studied.

García Barrón in her evaluation of the technical efficiency of the diabetes programme in units in San Luis de Potosí, Mexico[59] regarding the rating of the process indicator with inadequate results at 73.9%, because the variable that refers to the recording of laboratory tests in the clinical record obtained 65.4% as inadequate, and in less than 50.0% of the records a comprehensive physical examination of the patients was performed and an adequate diagnostic impression was not established. It also points out that other deficiencies identified are based on patient care in brief consultations, in which the doctor sometimes does not give precise indications that the patient must comply with in order to adhere to treatment; lack of resources for monitoring and control of the disease; lack of equipment necessary to perform glycosylated haemoglobin tests at the first level; elements that favour desertion and dissatisfaction of people with diabetes, all of which is reflected in the sustained increase in morbidity and mortality due to this pathology and its complications. [59]

In the research carried out on the postgraduate courses received on the subject of diabetic neuropathy in the last five years, the results obtained indicated that this subject had low priority in the continuing education plans of the teaching department of the Manuel Piti Fajardo Polyclinic in Santo Domingo, and that there was little participation by professionals in these courses.

Postgraduate courses are of vital importance because they provide basic and specialised training for university graduates. [62]

Regarding knowledge of the tools that can be used to evaluate neuropathic symptomatology in patients with diabetes, the physicians in the sample were totally unaware of them. We agree with Dr. Valero[63] who, in a study carried out in Maracaibo, Venezuela, states that the validated instruments for the detection of diabetic neuropathy are unknown to a large part of the doctors, which contributes to slowing down the correct diagnosis and adequate treatment, essential pillars in the control of diabetic neuropathy. This is an aspect on which we agree with Dr. Flores-Cuevas[49] who recognises that the lack of information among health personnel about these procedures and the importance of performing them increases the degree of under-diagnosis of the complication. Likewise, in the study carried out by Dr. Guzmán-Herrera[64] , when mentioning a validated and standardised questionnaire to be used in the diagnosis and follow-up of diabetic peripheral neuropathy, 90.3% of the total population mentioned not knowing any, while 9.7% reported knowing the instrument known as the Michigan Test.

There are multiple tools that currently exist that contribute to the diagnosis of diabetic neuropathy, even though the diagnosis is basically clinical and there is no need to perform electrophysiological studies by electromyography and/or nerve conduction velocity, when the history and physical findings are consistent with the diagnosis of painful diabetic neuropathy. [49]

Like any tool, these criteria do not replace clinical judgement but serve as a guide for the identification of neuropathic signs and symptoms. Hence the need for our clinicians to be familiar with them. However, there is no single tool that allows a comprehensive assessment of the wide range of symptoms. The combined use of different instruments together with an exhaustive interrogation and an adequate, structured and integrated physical examination, in the context of a comprehensive assessment of the patient, allows an early diagnosis to be made and consequently reduces the progression of the evolution of the different forms of neuropathy.

The literature related to the assessment of knowledge of diabetic neuropathy is abundant with regard to the patient; however, it is scarce with regard to the medical staff. Few studies describe the assessment of diabetic neuropathy knowledge in primary health care physicians.

In the health sector, the identification of learning needs and the search for new ways of training staff is one of the fundamental bases for the provision of services that are appropriate to meet the needs of the population. Given the large number of workers in the health system in the country, it is necessary to develop continuing education, which begins with the existence of a real problem or situation that leads to the identification of learning needs that generate the corresponding solutions. [56,65]

The identification by thematic nuclei of the expressed knowledge needs of professionals makes it possible to obtain more detailed information on the situation and provides the elements to be taken into account when designing courses or programmes for professional development. [65]

The first two thematic nuclei treated in our research were Generalities of Diabetic Neuropathy and Clinical Manifestations, in both of which unfavourable results were obtained. This is a worrying situation if we take into account that these elements constitute cornerstones for the doctor in order to make an adequate diagnosis and propose a therapy in accordance with the diagnosis. Among the professionals who participated in the study, we observed a high need for knowledge among both specialists and residents. On the other hand, the low identification of the main risk factor (prolonged hyperglycaemia) allows us to infer the low suspicion that doctors have for early diagnosis of diabetic neuropathy. We agree with the study carried out by Dr. Trinidad Escobar[58] on doctors attached to the Family Medicine Outpatient Clinic of UMF 11 on the diagnosis of diabetic neuropathy in Tapachula, Chiapas, which also reflects the lack of training in this area.

Another of the core areas addressed, where a great lack of knowledge was found, was that which deals with the Systems Affect of diabetic neuropathy, a central issue, because although symmetrical and distal polyneuropathy is the main form of presentation of this complication, autonomic manifestations (gastrointestinal, genitourinary and cardiovascular) occur in a considerable number of patients, and if not identified, they are associated with high morbidity, mortality and low compliance with treatment.

The diagnosis of diabetic neuropathy was the fourth core area evaluated in our study, where the worst results were obtained and where a poor command by the professionals was evident. Knowledge of this subject is of vital importance and should be present in all doctors when making a nosological diagnosis, in order to carry it out correctly according to the existing condition.

The greatest difficulties were related to the knowledge of physical examination techniques that allow for the detection of neuropathy, as well as the added value that professionals place on electrophysiological and imaging studies for the diagnosis of this complication, with clinical examination being irreplaceable for the early identification of neuropathic signs.

In relation to the elements indicated above in correspondence with what was evaluated in this study, we agree with Dr. Trinidad Escobar[58] as in his research he highlights the lack of preparation of doctors in terms of neuropathic involvement of the parasympathetic system, as well as in the fundamental aspects for detection and the use of the clinical method as the main weapon for making a timely diagnosis of this involvement.

The fifth thematic core evaluated in the research was the Treatment of Diabetic Neuropathy. The author considers this to be one of the most important core areas due to the implications for patients' health and quality of life of the appropriate choice of therapy. It is important to point out that inappropriate prescription is an important source of morbidity and mortality and is preventable.

When it comes to first-line treatment, we realise that this is perhaps one of the most disparate responses in our questionnaire, despite the fact that it has long been well established that the first-line treatment for diabetic neuropathy is tricyclic antidepressants, selective noradrenaline and serotonin reuptake inhibitors and α2y-calcium channel blockers (pregabalin). In this respect, these results correspond with the research of Dr. Trinidad Escobar[58] which highlights that among the doctors surveyed, a large group considers anticonvulsants to be the anticonvulsants of choice for the treatment of pain, despite the fact that these are considered by international guidelines to be the third line of treatment, which speaks of the lack of correct information in a significant proportion of doctors in the sample of this study.

However, it should be noted that in our study, as in the study carried out in Tapachula, Chiapas[58] , this lack of information is more accentuated in the resident doctors, while the majority of specialist doctors respond in a higher percentage of correct answers. In this respect, we agree with Dr. Guzmán-Herrera[64] in his research in a Family Medicine Unit, who considers that the misuse of drugs in the treatment of neuropathic pain is largely due to a lack of knowledge of the drugs of choice or first line as well as the correct doses.

In the final evaluation according to degree of specialisation, there were no significant variations in the results between residents and specialists, which indicates an equal lack of knowledge among all the doctors in the study, regardless of their degree of specialisation.

In our research, the highest percentage of professionals presented high learning needs, and therefore their knowledge of the topic in question was considered unsatisfactory. García Barrón[59] who mentions that at present there are still great deficiencies in offering quality care in the outpatient management of diabetes mellitus due to deficiencies in the training of doctors in outpatient care and the absence of a multidisciplinary approach to the management of its complications.

Despite the fact that there are not enough studies that evaluate the level of information among health professionals and that make it possible to substantiate the need for knowledge on this subject among primary care doctors, knowledge of diabetic neuropathy is a mandatory task for doctors, as adequate identification of the symptoms, the establishment of a timely diagnosis and, consequently, the orientation of effective therapy for patients who develop this complication of diabetes mellitus depend on it.

Although educational institutions have made significant progress in the training of health professionals, in the case of primary care, there are still insufficiencies in the knowledge and skills needed to respond to the demands of the population. It is essential that providers at this level develop skills such as the capacity for teamwork, communication, and a comprehensive and community-based approach to care, in order to deal appropriately with and solve the health problems that fall within their competence. [56]

It is widely accepted that continuing medical education is essential to enable health professionals to continue to acquire new medical skills and knowledge after their formal training has ended. In many countries, continuing medical education has been made mandatory for the continuing practice of health care and these include meetings, courses and workshops, specialised journal clubs, anatomoclinical sessions, and self-study through printed or internet-based materials. [66]

It is therefore necessary to focus more efforts of all health education institutions on training primary care physicians on the particularities of diabetic neuropathy. Training in itself represents the most important resource available to these institutions for the education and updating of their professionals. [67]

The results of this research provide elements for managers, health workers in particular, and agencies and organisations involved in the health of the population to take the necessary measures to eradicate the deficiencies detected.

On the other hand, it would be very useful, especially for primary health care, to extend the methodology used in this research to identify the impact of the diabetes education programme in other areas of the municipality and the province, as well as the deficiencies in its implementation that hinder the quality of care for diabetic patients and which in turn complicate the proper diagnosis and timely treatment of diabetic neuropathy.

The author considers that this study strengthens and can be the basis for the establishment of early detection programmes for diabetic neuropathy in our entity. It is imperative to develop training and improvement strategies in primary health care as a feasible alternative for dealing with diabetic neuropathy as a public health problem, based on the incorporation of professionals who contribute to the improvement of care with a comprehensive vision that allows us to address the physical, psychological, economic and socio-cultural aspects that have a decisive influence on the control of this chronic complication of diabetes mellitus.

7 CONCLUSIONS

An adequate approach to diabetic neuropathy is a hidden learning need for doctors at the Manuel Piti Fajardo polyclinic, and goes beyond being an individual need to become an administrative and social one, as it has a negative impact on the comprehensive care of diabetic patients. This results in a decrease in the timely detection of diabetes, largely due to the fact that diabetic patients are not followed up with the quality and frequency of consultations established by the programme. For this reason, the health area of Santo Domingo requires the immediate design of a professional development programme on diabetic neuropathy and the inclusion of all medical professionals, regardless of their degree of specialisation, in order to increase their competence, training and level of knowledge on the fundamental aspects related to the diagnosis and treatment of this complication of diabetes mellitus.

8 RECOMMENDATIONS

J Extend the study to the rest of the municipality's health areas.

J Design a professional development programme to reinforce the competence and level of knowledge of medical staff in primary health care, addressing fundamental elements for the early diagnosis and timely treatment of diabetic neuropathy.

9 BIBLIOGRAPHICAL REFERENCES

1- Naranjo Hernández Y. Diabetes mellitus: a challenge for public health. Faculty of Medical Sciences "Faustino Pérez Hernández". Sancti Spíritus, Cuba. Cuban Journal of Nursing 2016; 32(1). Available at: http://scielo.sld.cu

2- World Diabetes Report. World Health Organization 2016 WHO/NMH/NVI/16.3. Available at: www.who.int/diabetes/global-report.

3- Mendoza Romo MA, Padrón Salas A, Cossío Torres PE, Soria Orozco M. Global prevalence of type II diabetes mellitus and its relationship with the human development index. Pan American Journal of Public Health. 2018; 41: e103. doi: 10.26633/RPSP.2018.103.

4- Agreda JJO, Molina JRV, Pérez CDRP (2022). Analysis of diabetic peripheral neuropathy in type 2 diabetes mellitus in Latin America and the world. Mediciencias UTA, 6(2), 42-59 Available at: http ://revistas.uta. edu. ec

5- IDF Diabetes Atlas. Ninth edition 2019. atlas@idf. org Available at: www.diabetesatlas.org

6- Global Health Estimates 2016: Deathsby Cause, Age, Sex, by Country and by Region, 2000-2016. Geneva, World Health Organization; 2018. Available at: https://www.who.int/healthinfo/global burden disease/GHE2016

7- Pérez Jiménez D, Gámez Sánchez D. Current status of Diabetes Mellitus Mortality in the world and in Cuba. International Health Convention, Cuba Salud 2018. Available at: https://www.researchgate.net/publication/333308950

8- National Diabetes Statistics Report 2020: Estimates of diabetes and its burden in the United States. Available at: https ://www.cdc.gov/diabetes/data/statistics/statistics-report.html

9- ALAD Guidelines on the Diagnosis, Management and Treatment of Type 2 Diabetes Mellitus with Evidence-Based Medicine 2019 Edition. ISSN: 22486518

10- Diabetes Mellitus Report. CEVECE State Centre for Epidemiological Surveillance and Disease Control. 2019.

11- Kojdamanian Favetto V. (2022). NICE guideline 2022: update on the management of type 2 diabetes mellitus in adults. Evidence, Update In Ambulatory Practice, 25(2), e007015. Available at: https://doi.org/10.51987/evidencia.v25i3.7015

12- Cuba. Centro Nacional de Información de Ciencias Médicas. National Medical Library. Diabetes. World Statistics. Factográfico salud [Internet]. Available from: http ://files.sld. cu/bmn/ files/2019/06/factográfico - de-s alud-j unio - 2019

13- Domínguez Arnold Y, Licea Puig ME, Hernández Rodríguez J. Some notes on the epidemiology of type 1 diabetes mellitus. Cuban Journal of Public Health. 2018;44(3): e1127

14- Health Statistical Yearbook 2020. Cuba (2021) Available at: http://bvscuba. sld. cu/ anuario-estadistico-de-cuba

15- Annual Report on Chronic Diseases. Department of Municipal Statistics Santo Domingo. Villa Clara. 2020.

16- Rojas J, González R, Chávez M, Salazar J, Añez R, MD, Chacín M. Diabetes mellitus type 2, natural history of the disease, and the experience at the Centro de Investigaciones Endocrino Metabólicas "Dr. Félix Gómez". Diabetes International. Volume V. N° 1. Year 2013.
Available at: www.diabetesinternacional.com
https://www.researchgate.net/publication/263852357

17- Ortega Millán C. The other complications of diabetes mellitus. Diabetes practice. Update and skills in Primary Care. 2014;05(03):97- 144.

18- Chaviano Belette E, Somano Reyes AJ, Chaviano Belette HP, Hernández Méndez JL, La Rosa Macías OC. Diabetic neuropathy. Clinical and neurophysiological characterization in two health areas of Santa Clara. Medicentro 2005;9(2) 2277-6400-1-PB

19- Di Lorenzi R, Bruno L, Garau M, Javiel G, Ruiz Diaz ME. Prevalence of peripheral neuropathy in a Diabetes Unit. DOI: 10.26445/05.02.3 ORIGINAL ARTICLE. Rev. urug. med. interna. ISSN: 2393-6797 - June 2020 N°2: 17-27

20- Ramírez-López P, Acevedo Giles O, González Pedraza Avilés A. Diabetic neuropathy: frequency, risk factors and quality of life in patients at a primary care clinic. Archives of Family Medicine. Vol.19 (4) 105-111. October-December 2018

21- Cañarte-Baque GC, Neira-Escobar LC, Gárate-Campoverde MB, Samaniego-León LD, Andrade-Ponce SS. Diabetes as a severe condition presenting with typical complications. Dom. Sci., ISSN: 2477-8818 Vol. 5, No.1., Jan, 2019, pp. 160-198.
Available at: http://dx.doi.org/10.23857/dom.cien.pocaip.2019.vol.5.n.1.160- 198
URL : http ://dominiodelasciencias .com/ojs/index. php/en/index

22- Hodelín Maynard EH, Maynard Bermúdez RE, Maynard Bermúdez GI, Hodelín Carballo H. Chronic complications of type II diabetes mellitus in older adults. Scientific Information Journal. Volume 97 No. 3 May - June 2018. ISSN 1028-9933

23- Collective of Authors. National Diabetes Mellitus Programme. 1996

24- Barceló A, Karkashian CD, Duarte de Muñoz E. Atlas of Diabetes Education in Latin America and the Caribbean: Inventory of Programmes for people with Type 2 Diabetes. Division of Disease Prevention and Control. Non-communicable Diseases Programme. Pan American Health Organization, 2002. ISBN 92 75 07390 2.

25- Sotolongo Acosta MM, Fernández Bereau VB, Ramos Reyes AT. Educational program for the prevention and care of diabetes mellitus in students and workers of the University of Cienfuegos. Revista Conrado, 15(69), 19-25. Pedagogical journal of the University of Cienfuegos. 2019. | ISSN: 1990-8644 Available at:
http://conrado.ucf.edu.cu/index.php/conrado

26- Viteri Peñafiel DN, Lorenty Nolivos AA (2022). Diabetic Neuropathy. A Bibliographic Review. E-IDEA 4.0 Multidisciplinary Journal, 4(13), 92-101.
Available at: https://doi.org/10.53734/mj.vol4.id253

27- Sánchez Rivero Germán. History of diabetes. Gac Med Bol [Internet]. 2018 [cited 2022 Jul 23]; 30(2): 74-78. Available from:
http://www.scielo.org.bo/scielo.php?script=sci arttext&pid=S10122966200700

0200016&lng=en.

28- Hiriart M. The natural history of diabetes. Editora Huésped. Revista Ciencia. Vol 53. Num. 3 July-September 2002.
Available at: www.revistaciencia.amc.edu.mx

29- Turnes Antonio L. Introduction to the history of diabetes mellitus, from antiquity to the pre-insulin era. Sindicato Médico del Uruguay. 2019. Available in:
https ://www. smu. org.uy/dpmc/hmed/history/articles/diabetes melli.pdf

30- López D. A journey through the sweet history of diabetes. In Morales. J. (Ed) Diabetes 3rd Ed. Pachuca de Soto: Universidad Autónoma del Estado de Hidalgo. 2018. Available in:
https://repository. uaeh.edu.mx/bitstream/handle/123456789/11884

31- Guillén Núñez MDR, Araujo Navarrete ME, Duarte Vega M, Fonseca Soliz DI, Hernández Porras BC, Lara Solares A, Sánchez Mijangos JH (2023). Rational management of diabetic neuropathies: multidisciplinary expert consensus. Revista mexicana de anestesiología, 46(3), 184-190.
Available at: http://www.scielo.org.mx/scielo

32- Pérez Rodríguez A, Feria Pérez AC, Inclán Acosta A, Delgado Echezarreta J. Some up-to-date aspects on the diabetic polyneuropathy. MEDISAN [Internet]. 2022 Aug [cited 2022 Oct 04]; 26(4): e3855.
Available at: http://scielo.sld.cu/scielo

33- Ministry of Public Health. Guía de Práctica Clínica (GPC) de Diabetes mellitus tipo 2. First Edition Quito: Dirección Nacional de Normatización; 2018. Available at:
http://salud.gob.ec

34- Cedeño LA. Diabetic neuropathy from an updated pathophysiological approach. (2020) Available in: http://www.studo.com

35- Working Group of the Clinical Practice Guideline on Type 2 Diabetes. Clinical Practice Guideline on Type 2 Diabetes. Madrid: Plan Nacional para el SNS del MSC. Agencia de Evaluación de Tecnologías Sanitarias del País Vasco; 2008. Clinical Practice Guidelines in the NHS: OSTEBA N° 2006/08

36- Diabetes update guide. Definition, natural history and diagnostic criteria. 2018.

37- Standards of Care for Diabetes 2022 -ADA Guideline- La Escuelita Médica
Available at:
https://www.google.com/url?sa=t&source=web&rct=j&url=https://escuelitamed
ica.com/2022/03/21/standards-of-diabetes-attention-2022-guideline

38- A clinician's guide to type 2 diabetes: Recommendations from the GDPS network. 2022 ISBN: 978-84-944007-6-6-6

39- Vintimilla Molina J, Vintimilla Márquez M, Ordóñez Chacha R, Martínez Santander C, Montero Galarza G, Fares Orego X. Peripheral neuropathy of the lower limbs in patients with type 2 diabetes mellitus. Archivos Venezolanos de Farmacología y Terapéutica. Volume 39, number 1, 2020. Available at:
https://doi.org/10.5281/zenodo.4065015

40- Source G. Diabetic neuropathy. Offprint 2018 - Vol. 26 No. 2

41- Soria Iñiguez AB (2021). Advances in the diagnosis and therapeutic management of diabetic peripheral neuropathy. Available at: http://www.scielo.org.mx/scielo

42- Aguilar-Rebolledo F. Clinical guide "Diabetic Neuropathy" for physicians. Plasticity and Neurological Restoration. Vol. 4 Nos. 1-2 January-June, July-December 2005

43- Claudia Yáñez G. Confronting diabetic peripheral neuropathy in PHC. 2020. Available at: http://scielo.sld.cu

44- Aguilar-Rebolledo F. Diabetic neuropathy. Practical aspects, diagnostics, therapeutics and prophylactic measures. 2019.ISBN 978--607--7504--56-6

45- Ibarra Fernández R. (2022). Diabetic neuropathy: diagnosis and treatment. Available at: http://scielo.sld.cu

46- Rodríguez Arias OD, Rodríguez Almaguer F, Moreno Villalón MC, Reyes KL. Physical examination in comprehensive diabetes mellitus consultations. Journal Cubana de Endocrinología 2013;24(2):188-199. Available at: http://scielo.sld.cu

47- Quiñonez-Bastidas GN. Painful diabetic peripheral neuropathy and its diagnosis: an overview. Rev Med UAS. 2023;13(2):130-131. Available at: http://hospital.uas.edu.mx

48- Paredes EPM, Orantes LDC, Guerra JFE, Tanta JI (2023). Diabetic neuropathy in diabetic foot syndrome. Norte Médico, 2(6), 6-11. Available at: http://revistas.unc.edu.pe

49- Flores-Cuevas IJ, Cuevas-Núñez ZA, López-Ascencio R, Vásquez C. Detection of Peripheral Diabetic Neuropathy in Adults Over 60 Years of Age at the "Mexico BID" Health Center in Colima, Mexico. 2018. ISSN 16989465. Vol. 14 No. 4:1doi: 10.3823/1399 Available at: www.archivosdemedicina.com

50- Pedraza LC. Diabetic neuropathies. Clinical forms and diagnosis. [REV. MED. CLIN. CONDES - 2009; 20(5) 681 - 686].

51- Salinas Hernández LF, Bustamante Montes LP, Trujillo Condes VE, Cuellar Ramos CA. Diabetic neuropathy: pathophysiology, etiology and diagnosis. Revista de Medicina e Investigación UAE Méx / ISSN: 2594-0600 / Vol. 8 Núm. 1. January-June 2020 / pp. 8-16

52- Samper Bernal D, Monerris Tabasco MM, Homs Riera M, Soler Pedrola M. Etiology and management of painful diabetic neuropathy. Rev Soc Esp Dolor. 2010;17(6):286-296Guzmán-Herrera S, Muñoz-Zurita G, Pezzat-Zaid E.

53- Pérez-Guirola Y, Lombas-Rojas A, Cordero-Escobar I. Neuropathic pain in insulin-dependent diabetic patients. Rev Mex Anest. 2021; 44 (1): 51-54. Available at: https://dx.doi.org/10.35366/97777

54- Domínguez C, Flores C, Fuente G, García C, Giménez Rey M, Houssay S, Huber F, Santillán C, Urdaneta R. Update on the treatment of painful diabetic peripheral polyneuropathy 2015. Diabetic Neuropathy Committee. Argentinian Diabetes Society. Revista de la Sociedad Argentina de Diabetes Vol. 50 No. 1 April 2016: 35-46 ISSN 0325-5247 (print) ISSN 2346-9420 (online)

55- González García WA. Relationship of diabetic neuropathy and years of evolution in patients with type 2 diabetes less than 10 years of diagnosis (2022). Available at: http://ri-ng.uaq.mx/handle/123456789/3563

56- Sansó Soberats FJ. Twenty years of the Cuban model of family medicine. Rev Cubana Salud Púb [Internet]. 2005 [Cited 15 Jun 2021];31(2): [approx. 4 p]. Available at: http://bvs.sld.cu/revistas/mgi/vol20 5-6 04/mgi135 604.htm.

57- Aguillón de Ramírez DL, Ortega CE. Symmetric distal diabetic polyneuropathy in Unidad Médica de Soyapango September-November 2014. San Salvador. 2015. Available at: http://scielo.sld.cu

58- Trinidad Escobar I. Level of knowledge on the diagnosis of Diabetic Neuropathy by doctors assigned to the Family Medicine outpatient clinic of the UMF 11. Thesis for the title of Specialist in Family Medicine. 2022.

59- Garcia BA, Acosta RLP, Luna BE. Evaluation of the technical efficiency of the Diabetes programme in units in San Luis de Potosí. México. Rev Salud Publica Nutr.2012;13(3)

60- Casanova Moreno MC, Bayarre Vea HD, Navarro Despaigne DA, Sanabria Ramos G, Trasancos Delgado M. Guide to evaluate the diabetes education programme in Primary Health Care. Cuban Journal of General Comprehensive Medicine. 2014; 31(1):17-26

61- Casanova Moreno M, Bayarre Vea H, Navarro Despaigne D, Sanabria Ramos G, Trasancos Delgado M. Evaluation of the diabetes education programme in the elderly. Cuban Journal of General Comprehensive Medicine [Internet]. 2015 [cited 1 Oct 2023]; 31 (4). Available at: https://revmgi.sld.cu/index.php/mgi/article/view/82

62- Methodological workshop on professional development. Directorate of Postgraduate Education, Central University "Marta Abreu" of Las Villas. April, 2018.

63- Valero LK, Sánchez YE, López J. Venezuelan physician's information on diagnostic tests and treatment of diabetic polyneuropathy in Venezuela. Thesis to opt for the Title of Specialist in Family Medicine. 2019.

64- Guzmán Herrera S, Muñoz Zurita G, Pezzat Zaid E. Practical knowledge about diabetic neuropathy in family medicine specialists and residents of a Family Medicine Unit. Rev Biomed 2015; 26:5-11. Vol. 26, No. 1, January-April 2015. Available at: http://www.revbiomed.uady.mx/pdf/rb152612.pdf

65- Vidal Ledo M, Nolla Cao NE. Learning needs. Rev. Cubana Educ Med Super [Internet]. 2006 [Cited 15 Jun 2021];20(3): [approx. 3 p]. Available at: http://bvs.sld.cu/revistas/ems/vol20 03 06/ems12306.html

66- López Espinosa GJ, Lemus Lago ER, Valcárcel Izquierdo N, Torres Manresa OM. Professional development in health as a modality of postgraduate education. EDUMECENTRO 2019;11(1):202-217 ISSN 2077-2874 RNPS 2234. Available at: http://www.revedumecentro.sld.cu/

67- Casanova Moreno MC, Bayarre Vea HD, Sanabria Ramos G, Navarro Despaigne DA, Trasancos Delgado M. Design of a course on diabetes mellitus aimed at primary care professionals in Pinar del Río, 2016. Rev. Educ Méd. Sup. 2017;31(3): [approx. 9 p].

10 ANNEXES

Annex . Individual Patient Interview Guide.

PART ONE.

General data of the patient.

Age: ___ (Years)

Sex: Female ___ Male ___ Female ___ Male ___ Female ___ Male ___ Female ___
Male ___ Female ___ Male ___ Female ___ Male

Breed: White ___ Black ___

Smoking:

O Yes Number of cigarettes per day   Years of smoking

□   No Ex-smoker   Years of ex-smokingNever   smoked

Passive Smoking

Periodic ingestion of alcoholic beverages:

□   Yes

□   No

PART TWO.

The following questions are intended to identify the symptoms that you have experienced in relation to the different forms of diabetic neuropathy, so we ask for your cooperation and kindly ask you to answer the questions honestly.

1- Mark with an x if you have ever felt one or more of these symptoms in your feet or legs:

O Burn

Π Tingling or Burning

O Numbness

Π Pain

□ Needle prick sensation

2- Does the intensity of these symptoms increase during the night? Yes ___ No

3- Can you tell the difference between hot and cold water? Yes ___ No ___ Yes ___
No ___ Yes ___ No

4- Have you ever had the feeling that your feet are squeezed into a sock-like shape?
Yes ___ No ___ Yes ___ No ___ Yes ___ No ___ Yes ___ No ___ Yes ___ No

5- Have you ever had the sensation of losing your balance because your feet feel unsteady on your feet? Yes ___ No ___ Yes ___ No ___ Yes ___ No ___ Yes ___ No ___ Yes ___ No

6- Do you have difficulty getting up after sitting for a while because you feel weakness in your legs? Yes ___ No ___ Yes ___ No ___ No

7- Have you noticed a decrease in the strength of your hands with a tendency to drop objects? Yes ___ No ___ Yes ___ No ___ Yes ___ No ___ Yes ___ No ___ Yes ___ No

8- Do you have frequent hand tremors? Yes ___ No ___ Yes ___ No ___ Yes ___ No ___ No

9- Have you ever had injuries or wounds on your feet that you didn't notice until you

54

saw the presence of the injury or traces of blood on your socks?

Yes ___ No ___ Yes ___ No ___ Yes ___ No ___

10- Have your feet become hot, red or swollen without previous shock? Yes ___ No ___ Yes ___ No ___ No

11- Do you have any foot deformities? Yes ___ No ___ Yes ___ No ___ No

12- Do you have cracks or fissures in your feet? Yes ___ No ___ Yes ___ No ___ No

13- Have you ever had ulcers on your feet? Yes ___ No ___ Yes ___ No ___ Yes ___ No ___ No

14- Do you have dry skin on your lower limbs? Yes ___ No ___ No ___

15- Do you have increased sweating of the face and neck? Yes ___ No ___ No ___

16- Do you have a feeling of fullness or satiety after eating small amounts of food? Yes ___ No ___

17- Do you have difficulty swallowing food? Yes ___ No ___ Yes ___ No ___ Yes ___ No ___ Yes ___ No ___ Yes ___ No

18- Do you have nausea or vomiting after eating? Yes ___ No ___ No ___

19- Have you had episodes of diarrhoea mainly at night? Yes ___ No ___ Yes ___ No ___ No

20- Have you had any episodes of constipation? Yes ___ No ___ No ___

21- Have you ever experienced hypoglycaemia without symptoms? Yes ___ No ___

22- Have you experienced impotence or retrograde ejaculation during sexual intercourse? Yes ___ No ___ Yes ___ No ___ Yes ___ No ___ Yes ___ No ___ Yes ___ No

23- Have you experienced vaginal dryness during sexual intercourse?

Yes ___ No ___ Yes ___ No ___ Yes ___ No ___

24- When you urinate, do you have the feeling that you have not completely finished urinating? Yes ___ No ___

25- When you have an urge to urinate, are you unable to hold it back or do you leak involuntarily? Yes ___ No ___

26- Do you have repeated urinary tract infections? Yes ___ No ___ No ___

27- Do you have more urination at night than during the day? Yes ___ No ___

28- Do you experience palpitations when you are at rest?

Yes ___ No ___ Yes ___ No ___ Yes ___ No ___

29- Have you ever experienced dizziness or fainting when getting out of bed or standing up after sitting for a long period of time? Yes ___ No ___ Yes ___ No ___ Yes ___ No ___ Yes ___ No ___ Yes ___ No

30- Have you ever had a painless myocardial infarction? Yes ___ No

Specify with an (x) the time of evolution of these symptoms:

One year

∏ Between 1 and 3 years

∏ Between 3 and 5 years

O Over 5 years

Annex . Guide to Documentary Review of Individual Health Records.

Title of the study: Evaluation of diabetic patient care for the diagnosis and treatment of diabetic neuropathy.

<u>Individual patient records will be reviewed:</u>

Type of Diabetes Mellitus from which the patient suffers: Type I □ Type II □

Evolution of Diabetes Mellitus: (years)

Treatment of Diabetes Mellitus:

□   Hygienic-Dietetic.

O Hygienic Dietetics and Physical Activity.

∏ Hygienic Dietetics, Physical Activity and Pharmacotherapy.

Pharmacotherapy:

O Oral hypoglycaemic agents

O Insulin therapy

O Oral hypoglycaemic agents and insulin therapy

Comorbidities present in the patient:

O Arterial Hypertension

O Chronic Kidney Disease

O Ischaemic heart disease

O Dyslipidemias

∏ Obesity.

Frequency of controls in the last year: ___ Grounds ___ Consultations ___

Identification of risk factors for developing neuropathy from clinical history: Yes ___ No ___ Yes ___ No ___ Yes ___ No ___ No ___ No ___ No ___ No ___ No ___ No ___ No ___ No ___ No ___ No

Appropriate performance of the general, regional and apparatus physical examination: Yes ___ No ___ Yes ___ No ___ Yes ___ No ___

Performing a neurological physical examination with emphasis on:

Exploration of superficial and deep sensitivity: Yes ___ No ___ Yes ___ No ___ Yes ___ No ___ Yes ___ No ___ Yes ___ No ___ No

Examination of the osteotendinous reflexes: Yes ___ No ___

Lower limb trophism examination: Yes ___ No ___ Yes ___ No ___ Yes ___ No

Examination of the feet for lesions or ulcers: Yes ___ No ___ Yes ___ No

Appropriate interpretation of complementary tests related to the patient's metabolic control and to the type of neuropathy: Yes ___ No ___

Appropriate medical indications in relation to the type of neuropathy diagnosed: Yes ___ No ___ Yes ___ No ___ Yes ___ No ___ No

Time elapsed since the diagnosis of diabetic neuropathy was made:

O One year

∏ Between 1 and 3 years

□   Between 3 and 5 years

O Over 5 years

Annex . Questionnaire to professionals.

Dear Colleague:

The purpose of this questionnaire is to identify the knowledge needs on Diabetic Neuropathy of the doctors in the health area, and we therefore ask for your cooperation. Please answer the questions honestly. The information collected will only be used for scientific, research and training purposes. Your identity will be preserved and we will respect your decision not to cooperate with the research, if you so wish.

SECTION A.

Degree of specialisation:

O First Year Resident in General Comprehensive Medicine

∏ Second Year Resident in General Comprehensive Medicine

O Third Year Resident in General Comprehensive Medicine

□ Specialist in General Comprehensive Medicine

Have you participated in postgraduate courses received in the last five years on the subject of Diabetic Neuropathy? □ Yes □ No.

Which ones?

Are you aware of any instruments or tools used to assess the presence of diabetic neuropathy? □ Yes □ No.

If you answered yes, please mark with an (x) the tool you are familiar with:

□ The Michigan Neuropathy Screening Instrument (MNSI)

□ The Neuropathy Disability Score (NDS)

□   The Neuropathy Impairment Score in the Lower Limbs (NIS-LLs)

□   Quantitative Sensory Testing (QST)

□   Others, which ones?

Do you believe that the information you currently have about the diagnosis and treatment of diabetic neuropathy is...?

Updated. □ Yes □ No.

Outdated. □ Yes □ No.

Do you need more information about this complication? □ Yes □ No.

Are you satisfied with your current knowledge? □ Yes □ No.

Would you attend refresher courses on the subject? □ Yes □ No.

SECTION B.

1- Diabetes mellitus is characterised by a high predisposition to compromise microvascular territories; diabetic polyneuropathy is the most faithful display of this damage. Mark False (F) or True (V) for each statement as appropriate.

      In both type 1 and type 2 diabetes mellitus, the association between neuropathy and the onset of neuropathy is directly proportional to the age of the patient.

--- Hyperglycaemia is a primary relevant factor in the genesis of neuropathic involvement as well as oxidative stress and Protein Kinase C activation.

--- Diabetic neuropathy is most common in diabetics over the age of 50, rare in those under 30 and very rare in childhood.

Neuropathy affects sensory, motor and autonomic fibres of the central nervous system.

57

Risk factors include dyslipidaemia, high blood pressure, obesity and smoking.

2. The medical literature describes the clinical manifestations of diabetic neuropathy according to each of its forms of presentation. From the options below, select the grouping that best clinically characterises this chronic complication of diabetes mellitus.

a) Progressive pain, dysaesthesias, nocturnal paraesthesias, hypoaesthesia and abolition or decrease of the Achilles reflex.

b) Most important cause of diabetic foot ulceration and precedes Charcot neuroatropathy.

c) It is characterised by vascular claudication, dysautonomic signs (abnormal skin colour and temperature, sweating), depression and anxiety, sleep disorders.

d) Symptomatology prevails in the lower limbs with an asymmetrical distribution, manifesting as cramps, shooting pain and burning sensation with diurnal predominance as well as allodynia or hyperalgesia.

e) Neurogenic bladder, erectile dysfunction, gastroparesis and early satiety are some of the autonomic manifestations that are part of the clinical picture.

f) Diarrhoea is a late, daytime-predominant manifestation and requires a broad differential diagnosis.

g) Typical manifestations are described as "glove-sock" distribution, loss of vibratory sensation and impaired proprioception.

h) In later stages there is distal motor involvement with atrophy of the intrinsic foot muscles and the presence of ulcers as the ultimate expression of neuropathic involvement.

i) The most frequent electrocardiographic changes in these patients are decreased R-R variability and shortening of the QT interval.

□a,b,c,f,f,   g□d,e,g,h,   f□ a,c,e,g,   h□a,c,d,g,i □ None

3- Involvement of the autonomic nervous system is common, occurring in about 30% of patients with type 2 diabetes mellitus, and compromising the functioning of several systems and organs. Based on your knowledge of this topic, mark False (F) or True (T) for each statement as appropriate.

Autonomic neuropathy occurs in diabetics with less than 5 years of history and is usually correlated with the presence of distal sensory polyneuropathy.

Gastroparesis can run from asymptomatic to asymptomatic to vomiting and postprandial fullness leading to instability of glycaemic control.

At the level of the oesophagus, contrasted radiographic study may show mild dilatation, reduced primary peristaltic waves and decreased transit.

Silent myocardial infarction and sudden death are one of its most feared complications, but orthostatic hypotension is a late phenomenon.

Delayed pupillary reaction and anhidrosis are the most frequent clinical manifestations of this complication.

It is characterised by neurogenic bladder, erectile dysfunction and retrograde ejaculation in male diabetic patients and dyspareunia in premenopausal women.

Dryness, lack of skin trophism and alterations in the microcirculation (A-V shunt and lack of sympathetic response) play a major role in the development of the diabetic foot.

Nocturnal diarrhoea lasting hours or days, alternating with constipation, faecal incontinence and dysphagia are other characteristic symptoms of autonomic dysfunction.

4- Diabetic neuropathy is the most frequent and earliest complication of diabetes mellitus, yet it is the one that is diagnosed the latest. Mark (x) which of the following approaches allows an adequate diagnosis of this entity:

All patients should be assessed for distal symmetric polyneuropathy from the diagnosis of type 2 diabetes and five years after the diagnosis of type 1 diabetes and at least once a year.

In 60% of patients the diagnosis is clinical and the physical examination can detect neuropathy only with the use of Reflex Hammer, 128 Hz Tuning Fork and Semmens-Weinstein Monofilament.

The diagnosis of diabetic polyneuropathy requires the presence of at least one of the following criteria: typical symptoms such as burning, stabbing pain, cramps, numbness; alterations on physical examination of the thresholds of superficial and deep sensitivity and alterations of electrophysiological studies.

The differential diagnosis of diabetic neuropathy should be made with vasculitis, amyloidosis, HIV, chronic demyelinating neuropathy, and thiamine and pyridoxine deficiency.

Electromyogram and referral to a specialised diagnostic service   is   not necessary, except when there is a typical clinical course with predominantly motor involvement, symmetry of signs and symptoms and slow progression of the disease.

Peripheral nerve biopsy and skin biopsy assess fibre density at the intraepidermal level, as well as other histopathological features that allow a diagnosis with a higher degree of certainty.

Tests that assess cardiovascular reflexes such as the Valsalva Manoeuvre, taking the heart rate with deep breathing, and performing an electrocardiogram are the gold standard in the clinical diagnosis of cardiac dysautonomia.

Plain radiography is non-specific and contrasted studies show prolonged transit with variations in the intestinal lumen, dilated segments and thickening of the intestinal mucosa in patients with gastric dysfunction.

5. Once the diagnosis of diabetic polyneuropathy has been made, therapeutic intervention is required to modify the progression of this complication. Fill in the blanks with the treatment alternative in each case.

The   y   facilitate bladder emptying in
patients suffering from neurogenic bladder.

The   is a tricyclic antidepressant with a proven efficacy
clinical experience in the treatment of painful neuropathy.

The   is a fundamental pillar in preventing the progression of the neuropathic complications.

Gastroparesis improves with good management and with the use of prokinetics such as -   and   .

The treatment of choice for erectile/sexual dysfunction is based on the use of phosphodiesterase-5 inhibitors such as   and prostaglandins intracavernous.

Reduced dietary fibre and the use of broad-spectrum antimicrobials such as   .

The   is a modality of natural and traditional medicine which promotes the release of endogenous opioids in the spinal cord with favourable effects in the treatment of neuropathic pain.

Medicinal plant from which capscein is extracted for topical application and with proven effectiveness on neuropathic pain   .

Annex 5. Evaluation key of the questionnaire to professionals.

<u>**Scale based on 100 points:**</u>

Low knowledge needs: 90 to 100 points.

Average knowledge needs: 70 to 89 points.

High knowledge needs: Less than 70 points.

Questionnaire.

Question 1 = 20 marks (4 marks for marking each statement true or false correctly).

1- Diabetes mellitus is characterised by a high predisposition to compromise microvascular territories; diabetic polyneuropathy is the most faithful display of this damage. Mark False (F) or True (V) for each statement as appropriate.

-       -F-- In both type I Diabetes Mellitus and type II Diabetes Mellitus the association of neuropathy and the occurrence of neuropathy is directly proportional to the age of the patient.

-       V-- Hyperglycaemia is a primary factor in the genesis of neuropathic involvement as well as oxidative stress and Protein Kinase C activation.

-       V-- Diabetic neuropathy is most common in diabetics over the age of 50, rare in those under 30 and very rare in childhood.

--F--Neuropathy affects sensory, motor and autonomic fibres of the central nervous system.

--V---Risk factors include dyslipidaemia, high blood pressure, obesity and smoking.

Question 2 = 20 points by ticking the correct grouping of items.

2- The medical literature describes the clinical manifestations of diabetic neuropathy according to each of its forms of presentation. From the options below, select the grouping that best clinically characterises this chronic complication of Diabetes Mellitus.

a) Progressive pain, dysaesthesias, nocturnal paraesthesias, hypoaesthesia and abolition or decrease of the Achilles reflex.

b) Most important cause of diabetic foot ulceration and precedes Charcot neuroatropathy.

c) It is characterised by vascular claudication, dysautonomic signs (abnormal skin

60

colour and temperature, sweating), depression and anxiety, sleep disorders.

d) Symptomatology prevails in the lower limbs with an asymmetrical distribution, manifesting as cramps, shooting pain and burning sensation with diurnal predominance as well as allodynia or hyperalgesia.

e) Neurogenic bladder, erectile dysfunction, gastroparesis and early satiety are some of the autonomic manifestations that are part of the clinical picture.

f) Diarrhoea is a late, daytime-predominant manifestation and requires a broad differential diagnosis.

g) Typical manifestations are described as "glove-sock" distribution, loss of vibratory sensation and impaired proprioception.

h) In later stages there is distal motor involvement with atrophy of the intrinsic foot muscles and the presence of ulcers as the ultimate expression of neuropathic involvement.

i) The most frequent electrocardiographic changes in these patients are decreased R-R variability and shortening of the QT interval.

a, b,c,f,g,g U d,e,g,h,ₓ a,c,e,g,h a,c,d,g,i None

Question 3 = 20 marks (2.5 marks for marking each statement true or false correctly).

3- Involvement of the autonomic nervous system is common, occurring in about 30% of patients with type 2 diabetes mellitus, and compromising the functioning of several systems and organs. Based on your knowledge of this topic, mark False (F) or True (T) for each statement as appropriate.

---F Autonomic neuropathy occurs in diabetics with less than 5 years of history and is usually correlated with the presence of distal sensory polyneuropathy.

---V-- Gastroparesis can be asymptomatic to asymptomatic to vomiting and postprandial fullness leading to instability of glycaemic control.

V--- Nocturnal diarrhoea lasting hours or days, alternating with constipation, faecal incontinence and dysphagia are other characteristic symptoms of autonomic dysfunction.

---F--- At the level of the oesophagus the contrasted radiographic study may show mild dilatation, reduced primary peristaltic waves and decreased transit.

- --V--- Silent myocardial infarction and sudden death are one of its most feared complications, however, orthostatic hypotension is a late phenomenon.

- --F--- Delayed pupillary reaction and anhidrosis are the most frequent clinical manifestations of this complication.

V-- It is characterised by neurogenic bladder, erectile dysfunction and retrograde ejaculation in male diabetic patients and dyspareunia in premenopausal women.

- --V--- Dryness, lack of skin trophism and alterations in the microcirculation (A-V shunt and lack of sympathetic response) are of major importance in the development of the diabetic foot.

Question 4 = 20 points (4 points for each correct item).

4- Diabetic neuropathy is the most frequent and earliest complication of diabetes mellitus, yet it is the one that is diagnosed the latest. Indicate (x) which of the

following approaches allow an adequate diagnosis of this entity:

---x--- All patients should be assessed for distal symmetrical polyneuropathy from diagnosis of type 2 diabetes and five years after diagnosis of type 1 diabetes and at least annually.

x--- In 60% of patients the diagnosis is clinical and the physical examination allows the detection of neuropathy only with the use of Reflex Hammer, 128 Hz Tuning Fork and Monofilament.

The diagnosis of diabetic polyneuropathy requires the presence of at least one of the following criteria: typical symptoms such as burning, stabbing pain, cramps, numbness; alterations on physical examination of superficial and deep sensitivity thresholds and alterations in electrophysiological studies.

x--- The differential diagnosis of diabetic neuropathy should be made with vasculitis, amyloidosis, HIV, chronic demyelinating neuropathy, and thiamine and pyridoxine deficiency.

Electromyogram and referral to a specialised diagnostic service   is   not necessary, except when there is a typical clinical course with predominantly motor involvement, symmetry of signs and symptoms and slow progression of the disease.

x--- Peripheral nerve biopsy and skin biopsy assess fibre density at the intraepidermal level, as well as other histopathological features that allow a diagnosis with a higher degree of certainty.

 Tests that assess cardiovascular reflexes such as the Valsalva Manoeuvre, taking the heart rate with deep breathing, and performing an electrocardiogram are the gold standard in the clinical diagnosis of cardiac dysautonomia.

x--- Plain radiology is non-specific and contrasted studies show prolonged transit with variations in the intestinal lumen, dilated segments and thickening of the intestinal mucosa in patients with gastric dysfunction.

Question 5 = 20 points (2 points per item).

5. Once the diagnosis of diabetic polyneuropathy has been made, therapeutic intervention is required to modify the progression of this complication. Fill in the blanks with the treatment alternative in each case.

Cholinergic and alpha-blocking agents facilitate bladder emptying in patients with neurogenic bladder.

Amitriptyline/ imipramine is a tricyclic antidepressant with proven clinical efficacy in the treatment of painful neuropathy.

Metabolic control is a fundamental pillar to prevent the progression of neuropathic complications.

Gastroparesis improves with good control and with the use of prokinetics such as metoclopramide and **domperidone.**

The treatment of choice for erectile or sexual dysfunction is based on the use of phosphodiesterase-5 inhibitors such as **sildenafil** and intracavernous prostaglandins.

Reduced dietary fibre and the use of broad-spectrum antimicrobials such as **metronidazole** are essential for the treatment of diarrhoea.

Acupuncture is a natural and traditional medicine modality that promotes the release of endogenous opioids at the spinal cord level with favourable effects in the treatment of neuropathic pain.

Medicinal plant from which capscein is extracted for topical application and with proven effectiveness on neuropathic pain.

11 CHARTS AND GRAPHS

Table 1. Distribution of diabetic patients according to age and type of neuropathy.

Type of Neuropathy/Age		40-49		50-59		60-69		70 and over		Total	
		No.	%	No.	%	No.	%	No.	%	No.	%
Symmetrical polyneuropathy and		1	1,9	5	9,2	7	12,9	14	25,9	27	50,0
Autonomous	Cardiovascular	1	1,9	1	1,9	2	3,7	3	5,5	7	12,9
	Gastrointestinal	0	0	1	1,9	1	1,9	3	5,5	5	9,2
	Genitourinary	0	0	1	1,9	2	3,7	1	1,9	4	7,4
Mixed		1	1,9	1	1,9	3	5,5	6	11,1	11	20,4
Total		3	5,5	9	16,6	15	27,7	27	50,0	54	100

Table 2. Distribution of diabetic patients according to sex and type of neuropathy.

Type of Neuropathy/Sex		Female		Masculin		Total	
		No.	%	No.	%	No.	%
Symmetrical and distal polyneuropathy		17	31,5	10	18,5	27	50,0
Autonomica	Cardiovascular	5	9,2	2	3,7	7	12,9
	Gastrointestinal	3	5,5	2	3,7	5	9,2
	Genitourinary	2	3,7	2	3,7	4	7,4
Mixed		6	11,1	5	9,2	11	20,4
Total		33	61,1	21	38,9	54	100

Distribution of diabetic patients according to skin colour and type of neuropathy.

Type of Neuropathy/Colour of Bile		White		Non-white		Total	
		No.	%	No.	%	No.	%
Symmetrical polyneuropathy and		20	37,0	7	12,9	27	50,0
Autonomous	Cardiovascular	6	11,1	1	1,8	7	12,9
	Gastrointestinal	3	5,5	2	3,7	5	9,2
	Genitourinary	3	5,5	1	1,9	4	7,4
Mixed		9	16,6	2	3,7	11	20,4
Total		41	75,9	13	24,1	54	100

Distribution of diabetic patients according to smoking habits and type of neuropathy.

Type of Neuropathy/Habit of	Non-smoking		Former smoker		Passive smoking		Active smoker		Total	
	No.	%	No.	%	N	%	No	%	No	%
Symmetrical and distal	3	5,5	5	9,2	4	7,4	15	27,7	27	50,0

	polyneuropathy								
Autonomous	Cardiovascu	0	0	2	3,7	1	1,9	4	7,4	7	12,9
	Gastrointesti	1	1,9	1	1,9	1	1,9	2	3,7	5	9,2
	Genitourin	1	1,9	1	1,9	1	1,9	1	1,9	4	7,4
Mixed		4	7,4	2	3,7	1	1,9	4	7,4	11	20,4
Total		9	16,6	11	20,4	8	14,8	26	48,1	54	100

Distribution of diabetic patients according to consumption of alcoholic beverages and type of neuropathy.

Type of neuropathy/ alcohol consumption		Consume		Does not consume		Total	
		No.	%	No	%	No	%
Symmetrical and distal polyneuropathy		16	29,6	11	20,4	27	50,0
Autonomous	Cardiovascular	3	5,5	4	7,4	7	12,9
	Gastrointestinal	3	5,5	2	3,7	5	9,2
	Genitourinary	2	3,7	2	3,7	4	7,4
Mixed		5	9,2	6	11,1	11	20,4
Total		29	53,7	25	46,3	54	100

Table 6. Distribution of diabetic patients according to type of diabetes and type of diabetes.

neuropathy

Type of Neuropathy/ Type of Diabetes		Diabetes Mellitus type 1		Diabetes Mellitus type		Total	
		No.	%	No	%	No	%
Symmetrical polyneuropathy and		2	3,7	25	46,3	27	50,0
Autonomous	Cardiovascular	2	3,7	5	9,2	7	12,9
	Gastrointestinal	1	1,9	4	7,4	5	9,2
	Genitourinary	1	1,9	3	5,5	4	7,4
Mixed		1	1,9	10	18,5	11	20,4
Total		7	12,9	47	87,0	54	100

Table 7. Distribution of diabetic patients according to time of evolution of diabetcs and type of neuropathy.

Type of Xeuv' opatLT' time of diabetes progression		< Healthy		Eutre 5 -		Ende 10 -		>15		Total	
		No.	%	No	¾	No	%	No	%	No.	⅜
PoIiueuiOpatia symmetric and distai		3	5,5	4	7,4	Ll	20,4	9	16.6	27	50.0
>30шрu	CaidioAasciila	1	1.9	1	1,9	3	5,5	2	3,7	7	12,9
	Gastrointestinal	1	1.9	1	1,9	2	3,7	1	1.9	5	9,2
	Genitourinary	1	1.9	1	1,9	1	1,9	1	1.9	4	7,4

	No	%	No.	%	No.	%	No.	%	No .	%	No	%
Mixed	2	3,7	2	3,7	5	9,2			2	3,7	11	20,4
Total	S	14,8	9	16,6	22	40,7			15	27.8	54	LOO

Type of neuropathies / comorbidities	Symmetrical and distal polyneuropathy		Autonomous						Mixed		Total	
			Cardiovascular		Gastrointestinal		Genitourinary					
	No	%	No.	%	No.	%	No.	%	No .	%	No	%
Arterial Hypertension	10	18,5	3	5,5	1	1,9	1	1,9	7	12,9	22	40,7
Chronic Kidney Disease	2	3,7	1	1,9	1	1,9	1	1,9	0	0	5	9,2
Ischaemic Heart Disease	6	11,1	1	1,9	1	1,9	1	1,9	2	3,7	11	20,4
Dyslipidaemia	5	9,2	1	1,9	1	1,9	1	1,9	1	1,9	9	16.6
Obesity	4	7,4	1	1,9	1	1,9	0	0	1	1,9	7	12,9

Table 9. Distribution of diabetic patients according to metabolic control and type of neuropathy.

Type of neuropathy/metabolic control		Good		Acceptable		Malo		Total	
		No	%	No	%	No	%	No	%
Symmetrical and distal polyneuropathy		6	11,1	10	18,5	11	20,4	27	50,0
Autonomous	Cardiovascu	2	3,7	2	3,7	3	5,5	7	12,9
	Gastrointesti	1	1,9	2	3,7	2	3,7	5	9,2
	Genitourin	2	3,7	1	1,9	1	1,9	4	7,4
Mixed		2	3,7	4	7,4	5	9,2	11	20,4
Total		13	24,1	19	35,2	22	40,7	54	100

Adequate quality of follow-up and monitoring of diabetic patients.

Indicator	Result	Assessment criteria
Frequency of Consultations and Land	46,2	100
Anamnesis	68,5	100
Physical Examination	51,0	100
Indicated Laboratory Tests	80,0	100
Laboratory tests performed	52,0	90
Diagnostic Impression	49,1	90
Early diagnosis of diabetic neuropathy	33,0	100
Medical Indications	75,0	100
Medical thinking or judgement about risk of diabetic neuropathy	79,5	100

Distribution of doctors according to degree of specialisation.

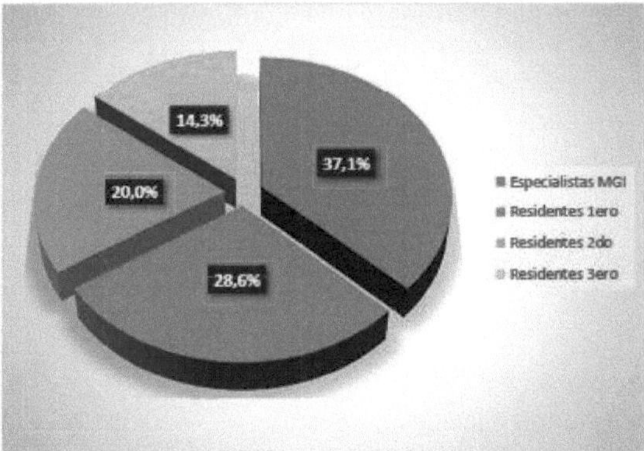

Table 11. Results of the final evaluation of professionals

Degree of Specialisation/Knowledge			Casualties		Stockings		High	
Needs			No.	%	No.	%	No.	%
MGI Residents		1st year	1	10,0	2	20,0	7	70,0
		Year 2	1	14,2	1	14,2	5	71,4
		Year 3	1	20,0	1	20,0	3	60,0
MGI specialists			2	15,3	3	23,0	8	61,5
Total			5	14,3	7	20,0	23	65,7

$$X^2 = 0,5637 \quad p= \quad 0,9970$$

Table 12. Knowledge needs of doctors about diabetic neuropathy according to thematic nuclei.

Core Themes* /Knowledge	Low		Stockings		Altas	
Needs	No.	%	No.	%	No.	%
1	3	8,6	6	17,1	26	74,3
2	4	11,4	9	25,7	22	62,9
3	5	14,3	5	14,3	25	71,4
4	3	8,6	5	14,3	27	77,1
5	5	14,3	8	22,8	22	62,9

$$X^2 = 3,8485 \quad p= \quad 0,8705$$

<u>**Legend: Thematic Nuclei ***</u>

1- General information on diabetic neuropathy.
2- Clinical Manifestations of Diabetic Neuropathy.
3- System involvement in diabetic neuropathy.
4- Diagnosis of Diabetic Neuropathy.
5- Treatment of diabetic neuropathy.

Table 13. Knowledge needs of MGI Specialists according to thematic nuclei.

Thematic Nuclei *	Knowledge needs of MGI Specialists (n=13)					
	Low		Stockings		Altas	
	N°	%	N°	%	N°	%
1	1	7,7	2	15,4	10	76,9
2	2	15,4	2	15,4	9	69,2
3	2	15,4	3	23,1	8	61,5
4	2	15,4	1	7,7	10	76,9
5	3	23,1	2	15,4	8	61,5

$$X^2 = 2,5384 \quad p= \quad 0,9599$$

Legend: Thematic Nuclei *

1. General information on diabetic neuropathy.
2. Clinical Manifestations of Diabetic Neuropathy.
3. System involvement in diabetic neuropathy.
4. Diagnosis of Diabetic Neuropathy.
5. Treatment of diabetic neuropathy.

Table 14. Knowledge needs of First Year Residents in the first year of the first year of

MGI according to thematic cores.

Thematic Nuclei *	Knowledge needs of First Year Residents (n=10)					
	Casualties		Stockings		Altas	
	N°	%	N°	%	N°	%
1	1	10,0	2	20,0	7	70,0
2	1	10,0	3	30,0	6	60,0
3	2	20,0	1	10,0	7	70,0
4	0	0	2	20,0	8	80,0
5	0	0	3	30,0	7	70,0

$$X^2 = 5.0584 \quad p = \quad 0.7513$$

Legend: Thematic Nuclei *

1. General information on diabetic neuropathy.
2. Clinical Manifestations of Diabetic Neuropathy.
3. System involvement in diabetic neuropathy.
4. Diagnosis of Diabetic Neuropathy.
5. Treatment of diabetic neuropathy.

Table 15. Knowledge needs of Second Year MGI Residents according to thematic nuclei.

Thematic Nuclei *	Knowledge needs of Second Year Residents (n=7)		
	Low	Stockings	Altas

	N°	%	N°	%	N°	%
1	1	14,3	1	14,3	5	71,4
2	1	14,3	2	28,6	4	57,1
3	0	0	1	14,3	6	85,7
4	0	0	1	14,3	6	85,7
5	1	14,3	2	28,6	4	57,1

$$X^2 = 3,6571 \quad p= \quad 0,8867$$

<u>**Legend:** **Thematic Nuclei ***</u>

1. General information on diabetic neuropathy.
2. Clinical Manifestations of Diabetic Neuropathy.
3. System involvement in diabetic neuropathy.
4. Diagnosis of Diabetic Neuropathy.
5. Treatment of diabetic neuropathy.

Table 16. Knowledge needs of Third Year MGI Residents according to thematic nuclei .

Thematic Nuclei *	Knowledge needs of Third Year Residents (n=5)					
	Casualties		Stockings		High	
	N°	%	N°	%	N°	%
1	0	0	1	20,0	4	80,0
2	0	0	2	40,0	3	60,0
3	1	20,0	0	0	4	80,0
4	1	20,0	1	20,0	3	60,0
5	1	20,0	1	20,0	3	60,0

$$X^2 = 3,6571 \quad p= \quad 0,8240$$

<u>**Legend:** **Thematic Nuclei ***</u>

1. General information on diabetic neuropathy.
2. Clinical Manifestations of Diabetic Neuropathy.
3. System involvement in diabetic neuropathy.
4. Diagnosis of Diabetic Neuropathy.
5. Treatment of diabetic neuropathy.

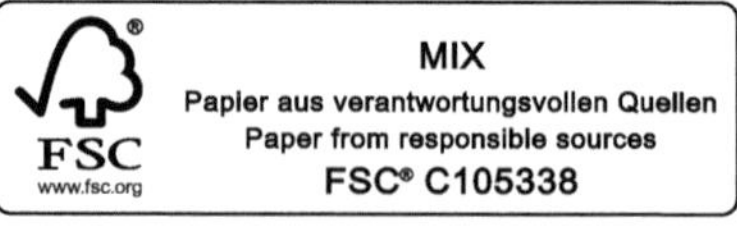

Printed by Books on Demand GmbH, Norderstedt / Germany